The
# BELLY FAT CURE™

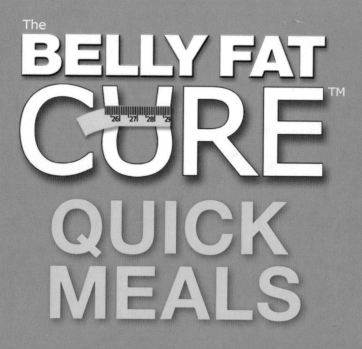

# QUICK
# MEALS

The

# BELLY FAT CURE™

## QUICK MEALS

Lose 4 to 9 lbs. a week
with on-the-go **CARB SWAPS**™

## JORGE CRUISE

**HAY HOUSE, INC.**
Carlsbad, California • New York City
London • Sydney • Johannesburg
Vancouver • Hong Kong • New Delhi

*To my dear friend and mentor,*
*Carol Brooks*

# Contents

*Welcome* . . . . . . . . . . . . . . . . . . . . . . . . . . xi

**1** Losing 4 to 9 lbs. with Quick Meals . . . . . . 1

**2** The One-Week Challenge and Beyond . . . . . 7

**3** On-the-Go CARB SWAPS™ . . . . . . . . . . . 15

**4** Sweeteners. . . . . . . . . . . . . . . . . . 231

**5** Ice Cream . . . . . . . . . . . . . . . . . . .239

**6** Soda . . . . . . . . . . . . . . . . . . . . . .247

**7** Bonus Chapter: Meal-Replacement Bars . . . .253

**8** Frequently Asked Questions (FAQs) . . . . .257

Index of Meals . . . . . . . . . . . . . . . . . . . . . . . . . 266
Acknowledgments . . . . . . . . . . . . . . . . . . . . . . . . 269
About the Author . . . . . . . . . . . . . . . . . . . . . . . . 271

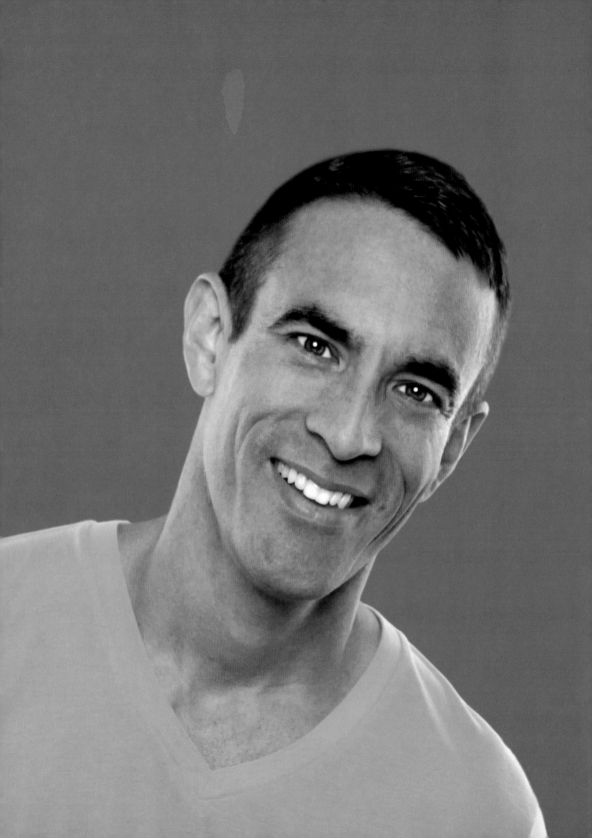

Dear Friend,

Do you frequently find yourself so busy that you eat a meal on the go and then feel guilty about it minutes later? You've been warned by the media about the many dangers of fast food, but the truth is, you can eat out and avoid the number one cause of belly fat: hidden sugar.

Today as a nation, we are busier than ever. I, like you, find myself eating on the run more often and want to be sure I don't sacrifice my health or expand my waistline in the process. I ventured out to fast-food chains, restaurants, and my grocery store's frozen-food aisle in search of the tastiest Belly Good meals. It is impossible to eat out and keep your waist small if you don't have a plan. Now I am able to share with you a new kind of CARB SWAP™ that follows the same principles that have helped millions of my clients lose weight on the Belly Fat Cure™. I call these quick and easy meals "on-the-go CARB SWAPS™." By avoiding the hidden sugar in meals you grab on the go, you can lose 4 to 9 lbs. a week.

I would love to hear about your success. Join me at **Facebook.com/JorgeCruise** and share your story!

Your coach,

*JORGE CRUISE*

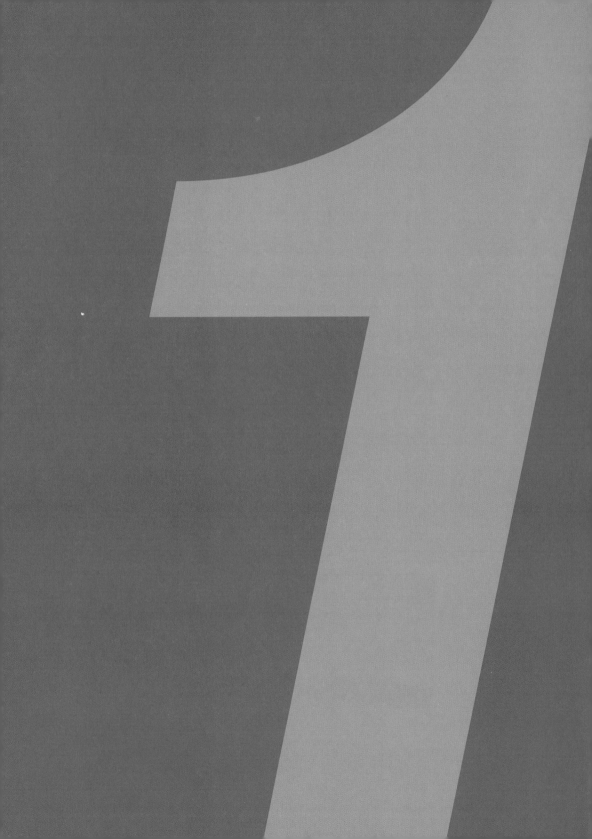

# 1

# Losing 4 to 9 lbs. with
# QUICK MEALS

## Lose Belly Fat in One Week

Time and time again you're told that eating out is a bad habit. Those same voices tell you it's expensive and unhealthy, and claim that the only way to be more attractive and gain confidence is to avoid dining out completely. Yet while these supposed experts argue against most fast-food chains, restaurants, and frozen foods, the truth is quite different. You can avoid the number one cause of belly fat—hidden sugar—while on the go. This book will guide you.

I created this all new, on-the-go edition because I know you lead a busy life. Above all else, my clients constantly tell me that they struggle to keep belly fat off due to their hectic lifestyles. No time, no time, no time . . . trust me, I understand completely. As the father of two young boys who is also dedicated to family and my mission, I understand what it's like to barely be able to find a free moment in the day.

Many Americans eat on the run out of necessity. Despite the messages we hear about the dangers of fast food, oftentimes we have no other choice. And as you already know, it's certainly not difficult to find. According to the National Restaurant Association, there are well over a quarter million fast-food restaurants in the United States.

## My Personal Struggle

When it comes to food, there's something to be said about the connection between convenience and comfort. There is a lure to fast food. Believe me, I'm not immune. I have fond memories of my mother taking me and my sister, Marta, to McDonald's as children. It tasted so good and always felt like a special occasion.

What wasn't so fun was being teased at school because I was overweight. As I grew up, I found myself depressed. I had low self-esteem and zero confidence. Physically, I had barely enough energy to meet the demands of each day. Fast-forward to my adult years. Not long ago, I was 40 lbs. overweight. I tried everything to lose weight: exercise, counting calories, various programs . . . only to fail over and over. I knew there had to be a better way.

There has been much research done on nutrition and fast food that discusses how calorie information posted on menus affects people's decisions about what to eat. You may have noticed that calorie counts are starting to appear on restaurant menus. However, **we cannot solve the rising obesity rate in this country by counting calories.** Nearly 70 percent of our nation is overweight, and that percentage isn't going to change just by posting calorie information on menus. Many of us—myself included—have tried to lose weight this way, and it has not worked.

My own lasting success with weight loss came when I learned that shedding pounds is not about eating less and exercising more. The true key to losing belly fat and keeping it off is simple: avoid hidden sugar.

## The Dangers of Belly Fat

Why should you be concerned about belly fat? It's about more than just looking good in your jeans. Belly fat is proven to be a contributor to three of the biggest killers in America: heart disease, cancer, and type 2 diabetes. In other words, you can literally gauge your life span by measuring your waistline.

As if disease isn't enough, the sugar that causes belly fat also contributes to aging. Sugar in your bloodstream can attach to the proteins there, creating modified compounds called advanced glycation end products, or AGEs. These compounds contribute to tissue deterioration and damage the collagen and elastin in your skin, proteins that are important for keeping your skin smooth and tight. In other words: more sugar causes more AGEs, which cause more wrinkles!

The number one reason for following the Belly Fat Cure™ : results. People consistently lose fat (often 4 to 9 lbs. in a week) and maintain a smaller waistline. The second reason goes hand-in-hand with the first: this program gives people the freedom to eat what they like while achieving those results.

I'm definitely a foodie—I love a variety of delicious, real foods. I also have a sweet tooth, and find myself eating chocolate on a regular basis. When it comes to my clients, I want them to enjoy great-tasting food and drop belly fat at the same time. I know from experience that it's impossible to stick to a weight-loss program if you don't enjoy what you're eating. The Belly Fat Cure™ remedies this problem through 15/6™, a simple system described in the next chapter.

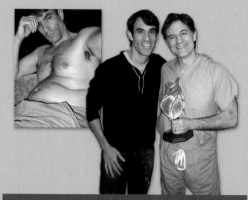

## Jorge lost 40 lbs.

Age: 40

Height: 6'0"

Belly Inches Lost: 5

Growing up, my best friend was food. I looked forward to hearing the ice-cream truck each day, and at night, I constantly begged my parents for second helpings of desserts. By the time I was a teen, my appendix burst and I almost died. It wasn't until I met Dr. Mehmet Oz that I was awakened to the fact that too much sugar was the heart of the problem and a significant contributor to belly fat.

My quest became satisfying my sweet tooth without all the hidden sugar. Because of this I was able to create the CARB SWAP™. I realized I didn't have to eat less or give up all the foods I loved—thank goodness!—in order to lose weight. Since then, it has become my passion to educate people on how they can lose weight and still eat the tasty foods they enjoy.

### BEST TIP FOR SUCCESS:

Never feel like you have to give up your sweet tooth. With my CARB SWAP™, you will always be able to find an option to keep you satisfied without eating less or feeling like you're dieting.

## UNDERSTANDING INSULIN

If you're not diabetic, you've probably never worried too much about your insulin. However, when it comes to losing weight, this hormone is crucial. Regardless of how many calories you consume or how much you exercise, without lowering insulin levels, you will never be able to lose weight. Why? Because insulin is one of the main regulators of fat cells.

Let me give you an example. When you drink a glass of apple juice, the simple sugars in that juice are released into your bloodstream. This triggers your pancreas to pump insulin into the blood. That insulin pushes fat into your cells, and more often than not, the fat zeros in on your waistline. Therefore, whenever you have a high level of insulin in your body, you are ensuring the creation and storage of more fat.

The solution to curing belly fat then, is to moderate your intake of sugar and carbs—even those from natural sources—to regulate insulin in your body.

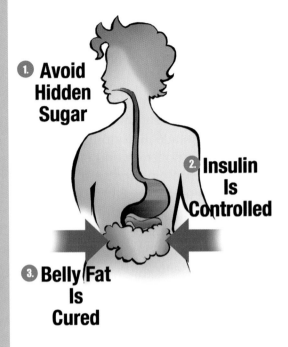

1. **Avoid Hidden Sugar**

2. **Insulin Is Controlled**

3. **Belly Fat Is Cured**

I personally love carbs. Honestly, I couldn't imagine life without them. That's why I created the Carb Swap System™—not the carb killer system! In my original *Belly Fat Cure*™ book, I provided hundreds of tasty CARB SWAP™ recipes to enjoy. In *Quick Meals,* all the same guidelines apply. This time, however, each Belly Good meal from a fast-food chain or restaurant, or available as a frozen entrée, is given a swap. Each Belly Bad meal in this book can be substituted by a Belly Good meal to help you drop belly fat. I call them on-the-go CARB SWAPS™. This is what I do to keep my own waistline in check: eat Belly Good carbs instead of the Belly Bad carbs I grew up consuming.

Identifying your belly-fat-curing options on the go is no easy task. That's why I've done the work for you. Now there's no need for you to struggle over what to order. This book is your road map. My most successful clients have lost 40, 60, and even 100 pounds because they were prepared. They had a plan.

As your coach, I want you to understand that eating out is not failing. There are many days when I'm caught between work and spending time with my family, and I need to grab a meal on the run. The key is knowing *what* to eat. If you rush into a restaurant in the middle of a busy day without knowing your options, it will be difficult to make the best choice. The information in this book will empower you to make positive choices next time you're out.

If you're ready to lose belly fat on the go, keep reading. This book will help you lose 4 to 9 lbs. in just a week.

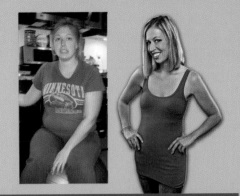

## Nicole lost 86 lbs.

Age: 32
Height: 5'3"
Belly Inches Lost: 15

After my second child was born, I ballooned up to 203 pounds. I tried to follow Weight Watchers a few times, but failed to lose all the weight or keep what I lost off. One day my dad gave me *The Belly Fat Cure*™, and I decided to give it a shot; 86 pounds and 15 inches later, I've finally found what truly works. I love all the quick options, and I especially love not counting points or calories!

Even the manager at my gym noticed the incredible change in my life. Not long ago, he pulled me aside and asked if I would share my story with other gym members. Now everyone at the gym has heard how the Belly Fat Cure™ transformed my body and increased my confidence. I've never felt better. This is my new way of life and I love it. Thank you so much!

### BEST TIP FOR SUCCESS:

Don't deprive yourself of a sweet treat at night.
I enjoy a glass of wine . . . guilt free!

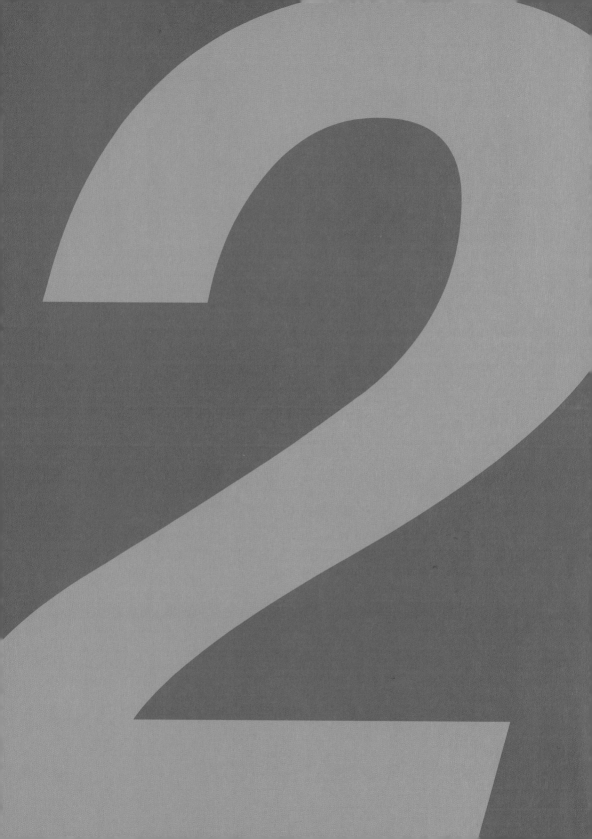

# 2

## The One-Week Challenge
# AND BEYOND

Many of my clients never imagined they could lose weight while still eating meals from fast-food chains and restaurants. They did not even consider that the foods they could have in order to lose weight would taste good! Yet with *The Belly Fat Cure*™ *Quick Meals,* both of these can become realities for you as well.

## How Quick Meals Works

To lose 4 to 9 lbs. a week, simply swap out the meals you're currently eating with the ones in this book. Here you will find tasty substitutions that are low in sugar and processed carbs, which can replace similar meals higher in sugar and carbs.

Forget about all the marketing and hype surrounding calorie counting. *Quick Meals* allows you to lose 4 to 9 lbs. a week by focusing on sugar and carbohydrates—not calories—because these are the main cause of belly fat. Many foods from fast-food chains and restaurants do contain a significant amount of calories, but more important, they can be loaded with hidden sugar.

## On-the-Go CARB SWAPS™

This book is based on my Carb Swap System™, the eating method I developed to guarantee that you know exactly what to eat. With the Carb Swap System™, you know just which foods you should steer clear of—those that are full of the sweeteners and excessive carbs that keep your insulin at a sky-high level, as well as keep your belly fat present. If you follow the Carb Swap System™, you will be sure that you always hit 15/6™ to transform your body.

Because all meals in this book are easily available while you're on the go, I consider each "Belly Good for Belly Bad" substitution to be an on-the-go CARB SWAP™. Every CARB SWAP™ in the following chapter is made by popular restaurants and brands that you enjoy. You already crave the taste of foods from your favorite chain—now all you have to do is find the foods that can help you stay on track every day.

## Insulin's Role and 15/6™

It is important to eat just the right amount of sugar and carbs each day in order to regulate the level of insulin in your body. Hidden sugar is the main enemy of a flat belly because of its relationship with insulin. If you have a high level of insulin in your body, you lock in belly fat. By regulating your insulin levels, you'll stop the fat storage process.

Based on my experience, I determined that you should consume no more than **15** grams of sugar and no more than **6** servings of carbohydrates each day to accelerate weight loss. I call this ratio the "Sugar/Carb Value," or S/C Value, and it forms the foundation of my 15/6™ system.

Servings of carbohydrates are calculated as follows:

- 0 to 4 grams of carbs = not counted
- 5 to 20 grams of carbs = 1 serving
- 21 to 40 grams of carbs = 2 servings
- 41 to 60 grams of carbs = 3 servings

## Nutrition Facts

Serving Size 1oz (28g/about 10 chips)
Servings Per Package 14

**Amount Per Serving**

**Calories** 160    Calories from Fat  80

% Daily Value*

| | |
|---|---|
| **Total Fat** 9g | **14%** |
| Saturated Fat 4g | **20%** |
| Trans Fat 0g | |
| **Cholesterol** 0mg | **0%** |
| **Sodium** 150mg | **6%** |
| **Total Carbohydrate** 17g | **6%** |
| Dietary Fiber 1g | **4%** |
| Sugars 0g | |
| **Protein** 2g | |

| | | | |
|---|---|---|---|
| Vitamin A | 0% | Vitamin C | 0% |
| Calcium | 2% | Iron | 2% |

*Percent Daily Values are based on a 2,000 calorie diet. Your daily values may be higher or lower depending on your calorie needs:

| | Calories: | 2,000 | 2,500 |
|---|---|---|---|
| Total Fat | Less Than | 65g | 80g |
| Saturated Fat | Less Than | 20g | 25g |
| Cholesterol | Less Than | 300mg | 300mg |
| Sodium | Less Than | 2,400mg | 2,400mg |
| Total Carbohydrate | | 300g | 375g |
| Dietary Fiber | | 25g | 30g |

Calories per gram:
Fat 9    •    Carbohydrate 4    •    Protein 4

Mission Tortilla Triangles
(10 chips)
S/C Value 0 / 1

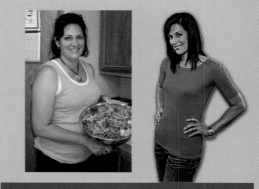

## Kellie lost 78 lbs.

Age: 39

Height: 5'10"

Belly Inches Lost: 8

As an adolescent, I was always the tall, skinny kid. But in my late teens I developed ulcerative colitis and had terrible eating habits. I battled the disease, and my weight, on and off throughout my 20s and 30s. After spending a week in the hospital with colitis symptoms (and having reached a staggering 225 lbs.), it finally dawned on me that I needed to change what I was eating.

I found the Belly Fat Cure™ and started slowly changing my eating habits. Now I've gone from being unhealthy and overweight to an energetic 39-year-old mother of two with a completely new way of life!

### BEST TIP FOR SUCCESS:

Commit to changing your life permanently. Eating 15/6™ and staying active shouldn't be temporary choices that come to an end in the near future. Once you get going, never stop!

# The
# BELLY FAT
# CURE™

## QUICK MEALS
## Agreement to Succeed

**I commit fully to putting myself first by following 15/6™ exactly in order to become a healthier, more confident person for myself and those I care about.**

**Current weight:** _____

**Goal weight 7 days from now:** _____

**Waistmeasurement*:** _____

**Goal waist measurement 7 days from now:** _____

**Your signature X**_____

*Join my Facebook page (www.Facebook.com/JorgeCruise) to receive my FREE video with Dr. Oz on how to properly measure your waistline.*

You won't have to worry about converting carb grams into servings if you're eating the meals featured in this book, because we've already calculated each S/C Value for you. But it is also easy to calculate it for a meal not found in this book. The S/C Value of any meal can be determined by consulting the meal's nutritional information provided on food labels and by restaurants. (See the example I provided on p. 9, from a bag of Mission Tortilla Chips.) However, many food labels and nutrition guides from restaurant chains don't provide the grams of sugar contained in the food. It is unfortunate that this crucial piece of nutritional information is often hidden from consumers. To assist you in overcoming this obstacle, I suggest you use my *Belly Fat Cure*™ *Sugar & Carb Counter,* which contains the S/C Value for thousands of items: hot dogs, fruit, salad dressings . . . you name it!

No matter where you find the necessary information needed to calculate a meal's S/C Value, you must aim for 15/6™ each and every day in order to be successful on this program. The good news is that this goal was specifically formed with busy people like you in mind. By this I mean that 15/6™

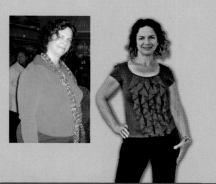

## Rosalie lost 85 lbs.

Age: 52
Height: 5'7"
Belly Inches Lost: 12

Not long ago, I was overweight and very unhappy about my appearance. My husband decided to make some diet changes with his friends and tried to encourage me to do the same. I told him, "I'll eat veggies and salads, but I'm still going to eat meat . . . and I'm not going on a diet." Around that same time, he saw a TV segment about *The Belly Fat Cure*™ book. He wanted to get it for me, but I said, "No, thanks." Well, he got it anyway. After ignoring the book for a few days, I finally decided to read it. I thought, *I can do this!* Needless to say, the results were incredible. I went from wearing a size 20 to a size 8. I can't say enough how great and healthy I feel!

I share my love for my new life with others every day on my blog, "The Belly Fat Cure™ PurpleRosy Style," found at **http://purplerosy.blogspot.com**.

### BEST TIP FOR SUCCESS:

Be ready to resist the temptation to cheat, especially around others. People will say, "Oh, one time is not going to hurt" or "You don't need to diet anymore." Be strong in those moments!

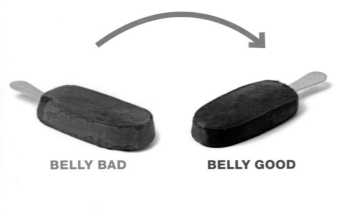

**BELLY BAD**     **BELLY GOOD**

is low enough so that you are able to rapidly flatten your belly, but not so low that you don't feel satisfied.

It is possible to stick to 15/6™ while still eating on the go. The media constantly tells us about how detrimental eating out can be for your body, and the majority of options at restaurant chains are indeed bad for your health. For example, marinara, teriyaki, and honey-based sauces are usually packed with sugar. Most low-fat dressings are high in sugar to try to make up for being low in flavor. And be cautious about seemingly healthy, high-sugar fruits and vegetables such as tomatoes and sweet corn. However, let me assure you that fast food *can* be healthy if you know what to look for.

When you have a little time to cook, feel free to use my original *Belly Fat Cure*™. You can substitute any of the Quick Meals suggested in this book with a CARB SWAP™ made in that book. It's just important to keep the S/C Value of 15/6™ in mind, both when you're eating out and when preparing a meal at home.

## Plan for Success

Join me at **Facebook.com/JorgeCruise** to get a free downloadable tracker to ensure that you're staying at 15/6™ each day. Although the calculations of the meals in this book have been done for you, I suggest you make it a habit to use your tracker each and every day.

If you ever feel like you hit a plateau on this program, I encourage you to use the tracker to make sure that you're truly sticking to 15/6™. Tracking what you eat helps you to stay accountable and ensures that you're eating exactly what you need to drop belly fat.

## Begin Today

Now that you understand both that eating out can be a healthy choice and that hidden sugar is the true cause of belly fat, you can begin to follow this program in your daily life.

If you want to lose 4 to 9 lbs. in one week, I encourage you to begin by signing the contract in this chapter. Promise yourself that you will *fully commit* to this program for one week. Display your signed contract on the refrigerator if you feel that will help you. It is critical that you hold yourself accountable, and it may even help you to have friends and family who support you to hold you accountable as well.

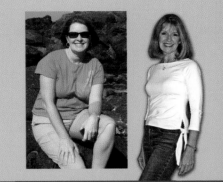

## Robin lost 40 lbs.

Age: *53*

Height: *5'8"*

Belly Inches Lost: *10*

Over the years my weight slowly increased. When I turned 53, I realized I was overweight and needed to do something about it. I read about *The Belly Fat Cure*™ in *The Costco Connection,* and the plan seemed very doable. I bought the book, and each day I watched the numbers on the scale get smaller and smaller.

Soon after, I attended one of Jorge's conferences in San Diego and learned about the Fast Track. Of course my friends thought I was crazy to eat all these delicious foods like cheese and bacon and expect to lose weight. But it worked! Now *they* follow the Belly Fat Cure™ and brag about it to their friends. It has been so much fun to go from a size 14 to a 6. Trust me, if I can do it, anyone can!

### BEST TIP FOR SUCCESS:

Stick with the plan and don't give up, because you *will* see results. Also, it's best to follow the program with a friend to help you stay motivated.

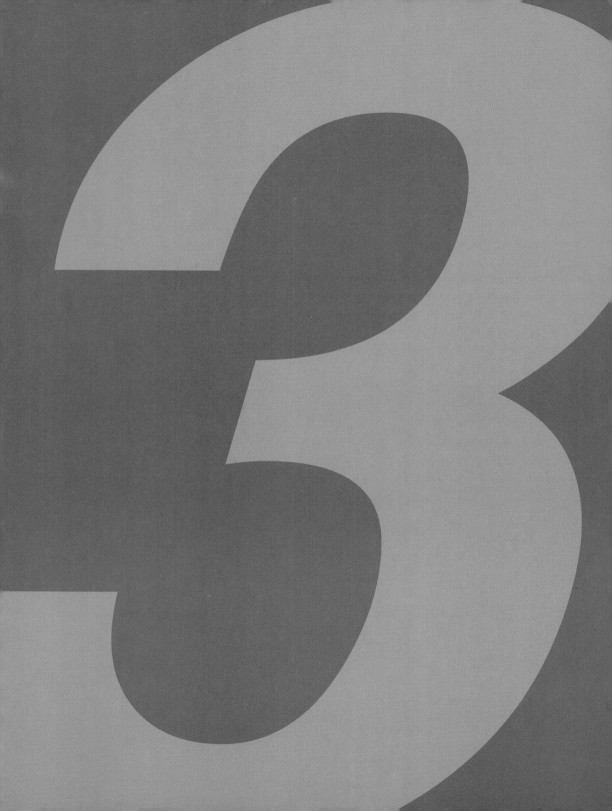

# 3 On-the-Go
# CARB SWAPS™

You're about to discover over a hundred on-the-go CARB SWAPS™ to help you easily lose belly fat. These satisfying meals don't require any preparation on your part, so you can quickly grab a bite during your hectic day while still sticking to 15/6™. (Keep in mind that each S/C Value in this chapter is based upon one serving size.)

Here, I have provided comparable meals from the same chain—one that is Belly Bad right next to one that is Belly Good. You'll be shocked to discover the frightening S/C Value of many of your favorite meals. These are the choices that have derailed your efforts to permanently drop belly fat in the past.

You will be pleasantly surprised by the values of the Belly Good options. You won't be stripping away all of a meal's flavor to make it a good choice. Instead, I'll show you how to keep it tasty but still Belly Fat Cure™–approved with a few easy switches. Sometimes all you need to do is order a meal in a slightly different way than it's listed on the menu to transform it from a Belly Bad option to a Belly Good one—usually, I note this with a few lines titled "how to order," so you'll know how to customize it "Coach Jorge style." (Note: It's important to be aware that restaurants and manufacturers often change their menus and recipes without notice, which could change a food's nutritional information, and thus, their S/C Value. If you can't find an item, or if the ingredients have changed, be mindful: the meal may no longer be Belly Good.)

Mix and match any of these three meals every day and see amazing results! If you choose to eat meals other than those recommended here, just remember to stick to 15/6™ and you'll be on track for a smaller waistline!

## Chili & Cornbread

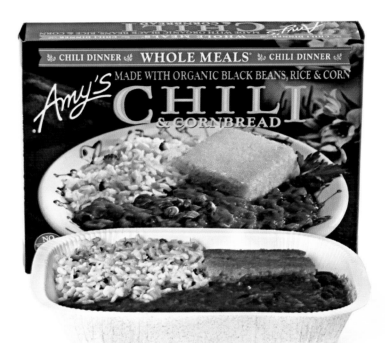

## BELLY BAD

**S/C Value = 14/3**

> This little box might do all right at a chili cook-off, but in my contest, it's disqualified for high-sugar content. Yessir, folks, keep this one on the red-checkered tablecloth.

# Vegetable Lasagna

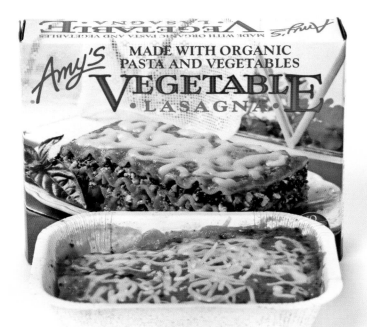

This Italian-inspired delight is dear to my heart: cheesy lasagna overflowing with flavor (insert gesture of me kissing the tips of my fingers and spreading them into the air)!

## BELLY GOOD

S/C Value = 2/2

## Indian Mattar Paneer

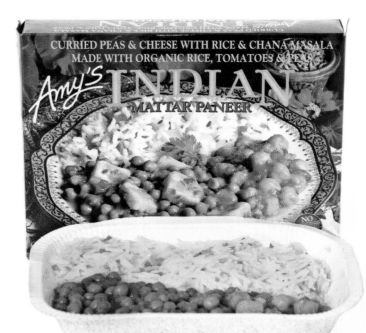

## BELLY BAD

S/C Value = 8/3

Okay, so you're getting a lot of rice and some measly vegetables . . . big deal. What else can you bring to the table, Amy?

# Indian Palak Paneer

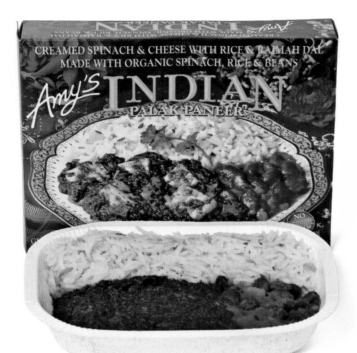

This pleasantly perfect paneer is nonstop delicious. Enjoy authentic Indian flavor with melt-in-your-mouth spinach and cheese together with red beans in ginger-garlic sauce.

## BELLY GOOD

S/C Value = 5/2

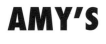

## Teriyaki Bowl

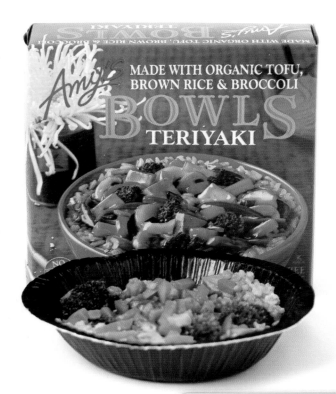

MADE WITH ORGANIC TOFU, BROWN RICE & BROCCOLI

BOWLS
TERIYAKI

## BELLY BAD

S/C Value = 15/3

This teriyaki bowl-a-thon is sponsored by hidden sugar—15 grams to be exact. But in the second frame I'm gonna pick up the spare with a delicious swap.

# Brown Rice, Black-Eyed Peas, and Veggies Bowl

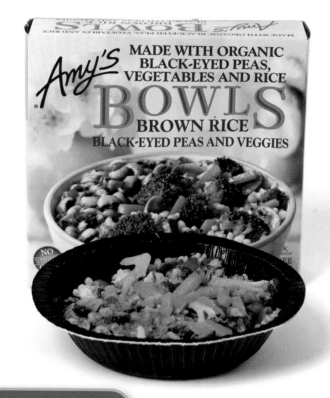

Here's one that will really bowl you over with flavor! Reach for the green box for tasty, vitamin-rich veggies and flavorful mushrooms over warm rice.

**BELLY GOOD**

S/C Value = 5/2

# APPLEBEE'S

## Mozzarella Sticks with Marinara Sauce

## BELLY BAD

S/C Value = 13/5

You may not realize this, but marinara sauce is almost always loaded with hidden sugar. Whatever the dish, it's always best to select a thicker, creamier sauce, for a much lower sugar value.

# Dynamite Shrimp

> **How to order:**
> "Hold the spicy sauce and bring a side of blue cheese." Also, consider sharing this meal with a friend to save yourself a carb serving.

## BELLY GOOD

S/C Value = 2/2

# APPLEBEE'S

## Paradise Chicken Salad

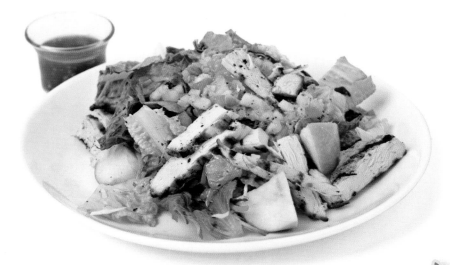

## BELLY BAD

S/C Value = 22/2

You may notice that this salad is endorsed by Weight Watchers, but don't let that confuse you: this meal does not cure belly fat. There are 22 grams of sugar in this salad! Let me introduce you to true paradise . . .

# Grilled Shrimp 'N Spinach Salad

Now here's a blissful match made in heaven that will have your waistline rejoicing. Indulge in delicious skewers of shrimp paired with steamed veggies and a spinach salad with ranch or blue cheese dressing. Plus, the S/C Value is divine.

## BELLY GOOD

S/C Value = 5/2

## Chicken Fried Steak

## BELLY BAD

S/C Value = 3/6

I'm pretty sure my belly fat went up a percentage by just looking at this picture. This county-fair all-star boasts 118 grams of carbs for a total of 6 servings. That's the biggest number in this entire book. Yikes!

# Asiago Peppercorn Steak

Tuck that napkin in your shirt collar cuz this is some good eatin'! Enjoy a thick cut of juicy steak with seasoned potatoes and fresh veggies! Yum!

## BELLY GOOD

S/C Value = 2/2

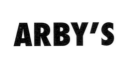
## Roast Turkey Ranch & Bacon Sandwich

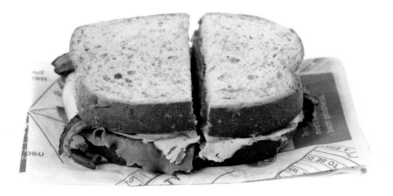

## BELLY BAD

S/C Value = 17/4

> All right, Mr. Arby (if that's your real name!) let's get real. Your sneaky little sandwich is packed with hidden sugar and will completely compromise my insulin levels. I disapprove.

# Prime-Cut Chicken Tenders
# with Chopped Side Salad

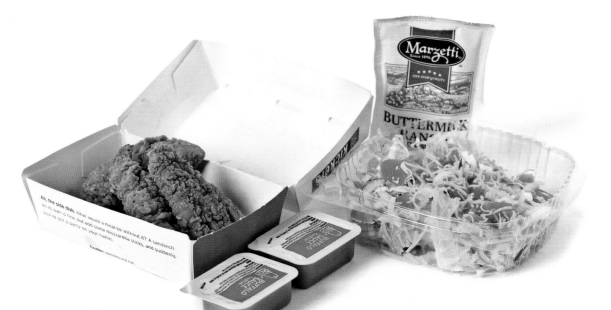

This tasty pair is one couple that has it all together: three golden-fried chicken strips with a cool chopped salad. How to order: "Buffalo sauce for the strips and ranch dressing, please."

## BELLY GOOD

S/C Value = 3/2

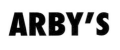

# ARBY'S

## Roast Turkey & Swiss Sandwich

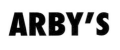

## BELLY BAD

S/C Value = 18/4

Brace yourself. This unassuming sandwich is about to make your waistline do a double take. Believe it or not, Arby's take on this classic pairing boasts a startling S/C Value.

# Jr. Chicken Sandwich with Chopped Side Salad

I feel like an Arby's matchmaker. Just look how cute this couple is together! Once again, the flavorful polarity of savory and fresh come together to cure belly fat with flare. How to order: "Ranch for the salad, but no tomatoes, please."

## BELLY GOOD

S/C Value = 5/2

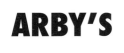

## Regular Beef 'n Cheddar

## BELLY BAD

S/C Value = 10/3

The carb value may not be intimidating, but 10 grams of sugar should knock your socks off. I've decided to rename this sandwich "Belly 'n Fat" with the tagline: "Beef up your waistline."

## Medium Roast Beef Sandwich

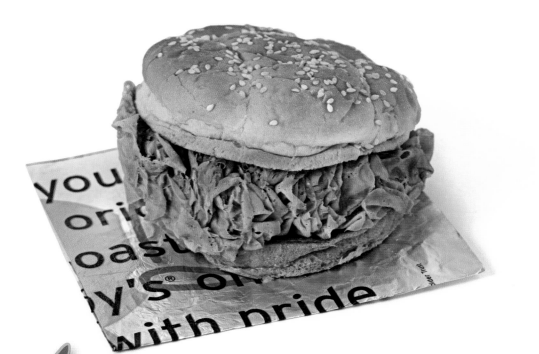

Medium by name, but extra-large on taste! Savory, thin-sliced roast beef on a sesame-seed bun and a tasty S/C Value. I want to reach through the page and take a giant bite!

**BELLY GOOD**

S/C Value = 5/2

# BOSTON MARKET

## Pastry Top
## Chicken Pot Pie

## BELLY BAD

S/C Value = 6/3

Look at this flying saucer of carbs. Area 51 might want to know that they're missing a specimen. Honestly, the last thing you want is this UFO hovering over your waistline.

# Turkey Breast, Mashed Potatoes, and Spinach

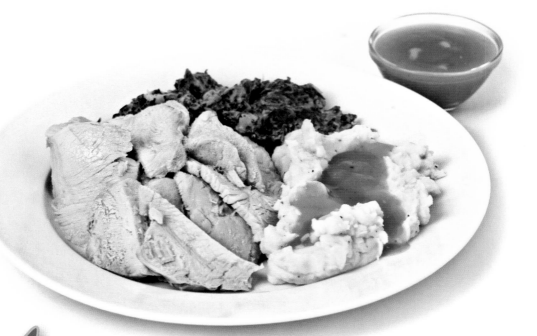

It's time to give thanks! Celebrate your belly-fat-dropping freedom with thick slices of delicious turkey and mashed potatoes with gravy. How to order: "Only half a serving of mashed potatoes, please."

## BELLY GOOD

S/C Value = 2/2

# BOSTON MARKET

## Mediterranean Salad with Cornbread

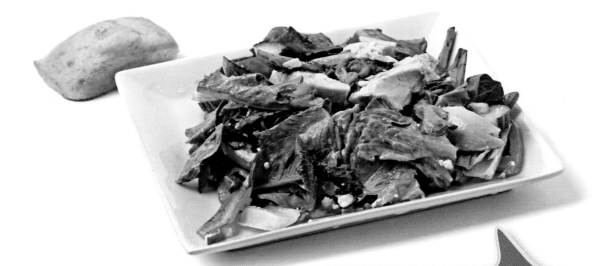

## BELLY BAD

S/C Value = 21/4

What do you get when you combine colonial sensibility with Middle Eastern cuisine? A geographically confused meal with a hidden-sugar value of international proportions. Keep this stamp off your passport.

# Chicken Breast with Garlic Dill New Potatoes and Chicken Tortilla Soup

The Market allows you to blend together another couple cuisines here, but this time pulls it off: thick slices of all-white chicken, garlic dill potatoes, and a scrumptious tortilla soup. How to order: "No tortilla strips on the soup."

## BELLY GOOD

S/C Value = 5/2

# BOSTON MARKET

## Meatloaf, Vegetable Stuffing, and Macaroni and Cheese

## BELLY BAD

S/C Value = 13/5

This meatloaf masquerades as homegrown goodness only to tip the bathroom scale with some heavy numbers. Better to keep this meal in the pan than kick it loosen-the-belt style.

# Brisket, Garlicky Lemon Spinach, and Loaded Mashed Potatoes

Pull up a front seat to this plate of Boston Market magic: delectable brisket; loaded mashed potatoes with cheddar cheese, bacon bits, and butter; and garlic-seasoned spinach. My foodie heart just skipped a beat!

## BELLY GOOD

S/C Value = 5/2

# BURGER KING

## BK Breakfast Ciabatta Club Sandwich

## BELLY BAD

S/C Value = 9/3

If you want to "have it your way," be sure to avoid this early-morning malfunction. I promise, you don't want to be a member of this breakfast club.

# Sausage, Egg & Cheese Croissan'wich, and Coffee with Cream

## BELLY GOOD

S/C Value = 5/2

You know you're King when you can make up new words to describe your food. Despite the fact that "Croissan'wich" isn't in the dictionary, this CARB SWAP™ is a great way to say "rise and shine."

# BURGER KING

## 5 Piece French Toast Sticks with Syrup

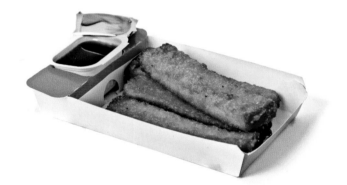

## BELLY BAD

S/C Value = 30/4

This sugary, deep-fried breakfast novelty is far from a sweet deal for your waistline. Rather than starting your day with the French, let's try a Latin approach . . .

# Breakfast Burrito with Sausage, Egg, Cheese & Salsa, and Regular Iced Coffee with Cream

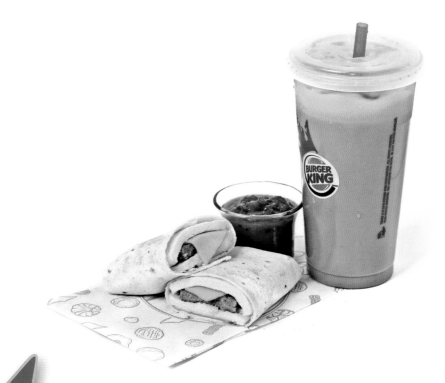

Bite into this toasty breakfast favorite for savory sausage, egg, and melted cheese wrapped together in a warm tortilla with salsa. Add iced coffee with cream for a perfect match.

## BELLY GOOD

S/C Value = 2/2

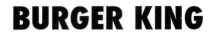

# BURGER KING

## Tendercrisp Garden Salad, with Fat-Free Ranch Dressing

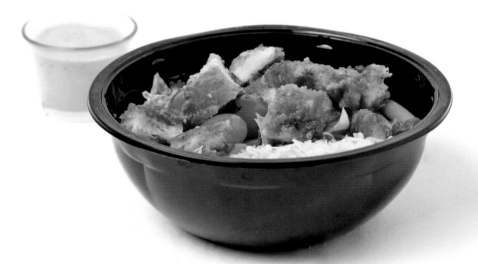

## BELLY BAD

S/C Value = 10/3

This crispy chicken salad is all show. Oh, it might appear healthy, but its true character is loaded with hidden sugar. The culprits? Breaded chicken and fat-free ranch.

# Tendergrill Garden Salad, with Ranch Dressing

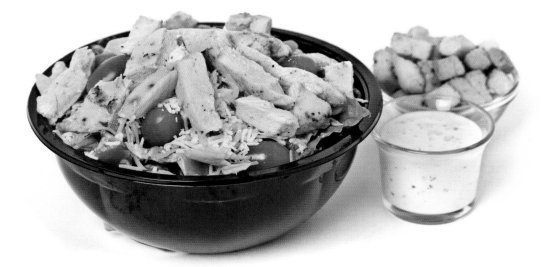

Talk about grilling the competition. If the fat-blasting S/C Value doesn't win your heart, the side of croutons certainly will. How to order: "I'll have the Tendergrill Garden Salad with ranch (not fat free)." Believe it or not, "fat free" in this case adds 4 additional grams of sugar per serving.

## BELLY GOOD

S/C Value = 5/1

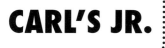

# CARL'S JR.

## Low-Carb
## Teriyaki Burger

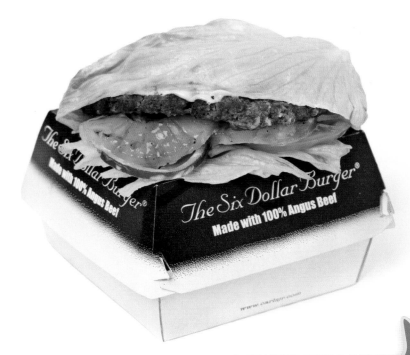

## BELLY BAD

S/C Value = 18/1

Only one of these low-carb options hits the mark. I'll break the suspense for you: it's not this one. This heavy hitter throws a sugary one-two combo of teriyaki sauce and grilled pineapple.

# Low-Carb Portobello Burger

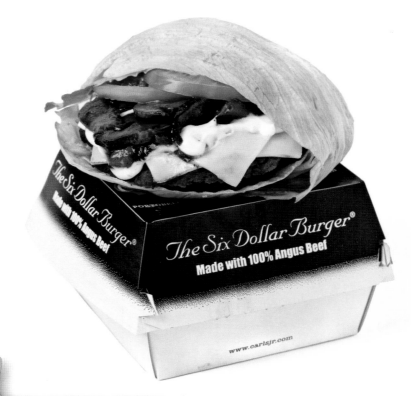

My hat is off to Sir Carl for keeping sugar out and taste in. This scrumptious burger brings it: juicy beef and melted Swiss topped with savory mushrooms.

## BELLY GOOD

S/C Value = 5/1

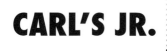

# CARL'S JR.

## Charbroiled BBQ Chicken Sandwich

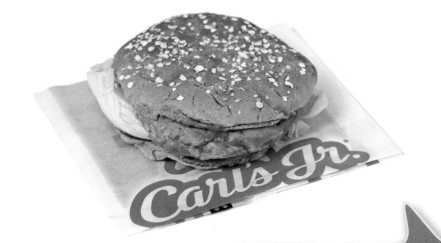

## BELLY BAD

S/C Value = 13/3

I think to say "Jr." is a bit of a stretch here. This modestly sized sandwich is ready to make a huge contribution to your waistline. Do yourself a big favor and say "no thanks" to 13 grams of hidden sugar.

# 5 Piece Hand-Breaded
# Chicken Tenders with Side Salad

I love tasty combos! Let's break it down: golden-fried chicken tenders with a fresh salad loaded with crisp lettuce and lip-smacking blue cheese dressing (but be sure to pass on the dipping sauces, which are loaded with sugar). Wash it all down with a sweet Vitamin Water Zero.

## BELLY GOOD

S/C Value = 4/2

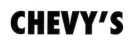

# CHEVY'S

## Grilled Fajita Salad

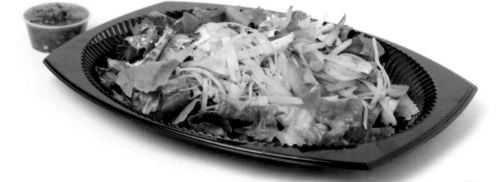

## BELLY BAD

S/C Value = 31/4

> If I were a matador, I would use my cape as a red flag. I'd rather take my chances with the bull than this salad. Sure, it may not look intimidating, but then it lowers its sugary horns and charges after your pancreas.

# Grilled Chicken Salad

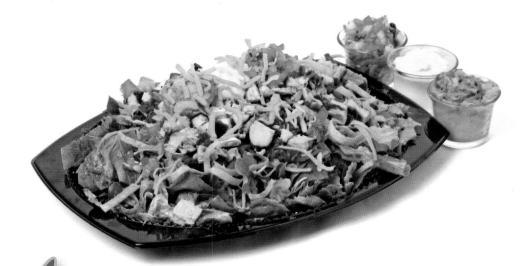

Bust out the sombrero and celebrate a Mexican salad done right! This taste-sensation has a festive lineup: seasoned chicken, rich guacamole, sour cream, and pico de gallo, all piled high on crisp greens. Olé!

## BELLY GOOD

S/C Value = 5/2

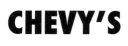

# CHEVY'S

## Lunch Value Carnitas

## BELLY BAD

S/C Value = 16/3

Even *without* rice and guacamole, this lunch still slow roasts my belly-fat-cure expectations. Leave this carnivorous, high-sugar combo in the roaster, mis amigos.

# Lunch Value Original
# Famous Chicken Fajitas

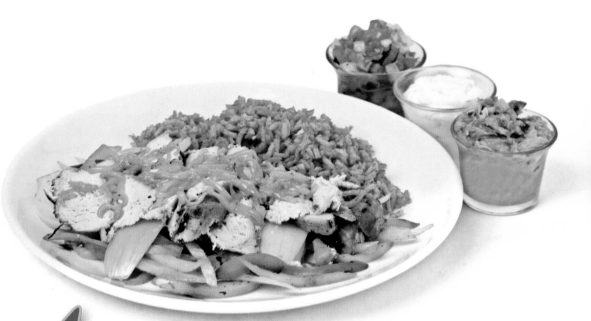

Holy guacamole, now *this* is how you do fajitas! With all this good stuff, there's really only one other thing you need to know . . . how to order: "No beans, please, and hold the sweet corn."

## BELLY GOOD

S/C Value = 4/2

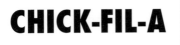

# CHICK-FIL-A

## Yogurt Parfait with Granola

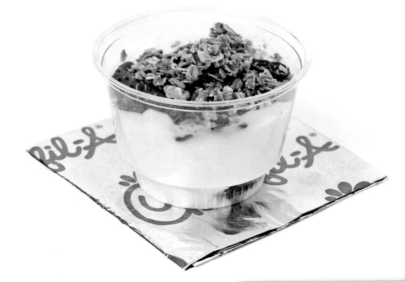

## BELLY BAD

S/C Value = 39/3

Aha! This sultry parfait is flirting with your healthy preconceptions. Oh, it'll try to seduce you with fruit and granola, but the truth is that both of these (as well as the yogurt) are loaded with sugar.

# Sausage Breakfast Burrito

"Move over, parfait,
I've got belly fat to cure!"
That's right! You won't regret
this sizzling breakfast bonanza
of seasoned sausage, melted
cheese, and spicy salsa for
more taste and a smaller waist.

## BELLY GOOD

S/C Value = 3/2

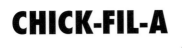

# CHICK-FIL-A

## Chargrilled & Fruit Salad

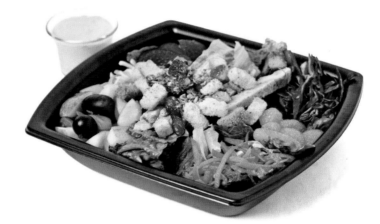

## BELLY BAD

S/C Value = 17/2

A friendly reminder from your coach: fruit is sugar. And by the way, sugar grams aren't like rollover minutes. Just because you only had 10 grams of sugar yesterday, that doesn't mean you can have 20 today.

# Southwest Chargrilled Salad with a Half Order of Waffle Fries

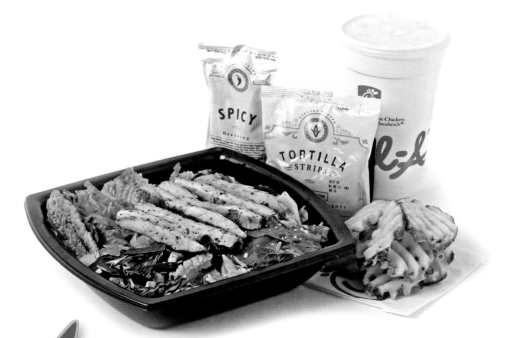

"Jorge, are those fries?!" Absolutely! Just remember two simple guidelines to keep your taste buds and waistline happy: "No tomatoes on the salad, and only a half order of waffle fries."

## BELLY GOOD

S/C Value = 5/2

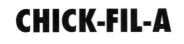

## Chicken-Salad Sandwich

## BELLY BAD

S/C Value = 12/3

Peek-a-boo, I found you! This classic sandwich is a favorite hiding place for sugar. Not all chicken is created equal, especially when the original white meat is in salad form.

# 3 Piece Chick-n-Strips with Hearty Breast of Chicken Soup

Mmm, I heart this CARB SWAP™.
Enjoy tasty strips of fried chicken with a side of mayo for dipping and a savory side of chicken soup for an exceptional S/C Value.

## BELLY GOOD

S/C Value = 5/2

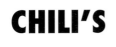

# Baby Back Ribs

## BELLY BAD

S/C Value = 14/4

I'm gonna change up the jingle a bit: "I want my belly back, belly back, belly back . . . " Sorry to say it, team, but this Chili's staple is layered with sugary barbeque sauce and making a beeline for your waistline.

# Classic Sirloin, and Spicy Garlic & Lime Grilled Shrimp

I wish this book was a scratch 'n' sniff. For now, just imagine the savory aroma of juicy steak and succulent shrimp, hot off the grill and dripping with butter.

**BELLY GOOD**

S/C Value = 1/2

## Caribbean Salad
## with Chicken

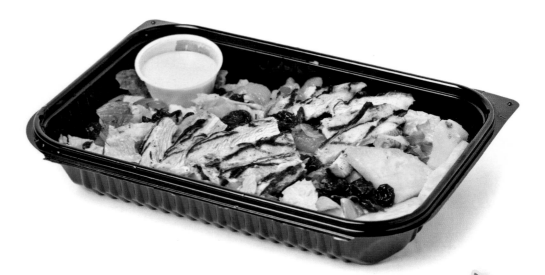

## BELLY BAD

S/C Value = 50/4

"X" definitely marks the spot on this sugary treasure map . . . and it's right on your belly. Order this salad and you'll consume more than three days' worth of sugar faster than you can say "SPF."

# Grilled Salmon with Garlic & Herbs

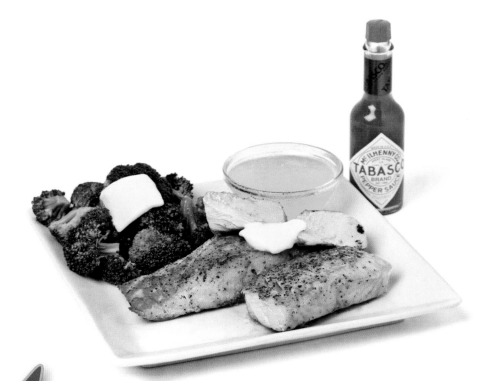

Let down your anchor in the clear, S/C Value waters of this sensational swap. Dive into flavorful, flaky salmon seasoned with garlic and herbs, along with a tasty side of broccoli topped with melted butter.

## BELLY GOOD

S/C Value = 1/2

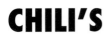

# CHILI'S

## Bacon Ranch Quesadilla

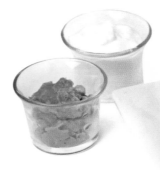

## BELLY BAD

S/C Value = 6/5

Saddle up, partner, it's time to corral the carbs. You might find your waistline singing "Kumbaya" 'round the campfire to redeem all 5 servings. Tarnation!

# Chicken Fajitas

Y'all ready for some seriously good eats?! Grab a fork and dig in to hot strips of chicken stacked on grilled peppers with guacamole, sour cream, and cheese. How to order: "Only one tortilla, please!"

## BELLY GOOD

S/C Value = 5/2

## Veggie Bowl

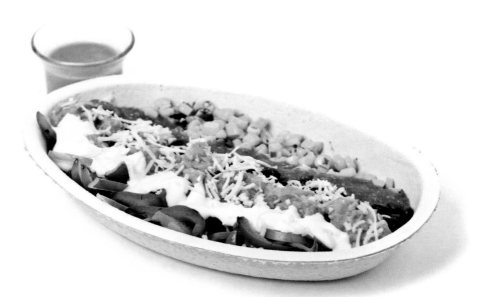

## BELLY BAD

S/C Value = 25/5

Customizing your veggie bowl like *this* will shatter your belly-fat-losing dreams like a sweet-toothed niño swinging for the fences to bust open a piñata. The vinaigrette alone contributes 11 grams of sugar to the total.

# Vegetarian Burrito Bowl

Chipotle's build-your-own style makes it simple. How to order: "I'll have a veggie bowl with rice, a half-serving of pinto beans, fajita veggies, salsa [take your pick], sour cream, cheese, and guacamole."

## BELLY GOOD

S/C Value = 5/2

# CHIPOTLE

## Salad

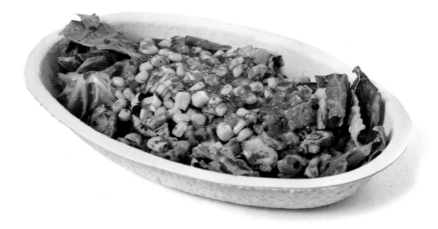

## BELLY BAD

S/C Value = 20/5

This seemingly innocent plate of fresh greens is actually a special-ops hideout for sugar. Don't surrender a smaller waist to this platoon of vinaigrette and corn salsa when there's a better choice.

## Salad

How to order:
"I'll have a salad with black beans, chicken, fresh tomato salsa, cheese, and avocado."
Goodness, my stomach just growled . . .

## BELLY GOOD

S/C Value = 5/2

# CHIPOTLE

## Tacos with Flour Tortillas

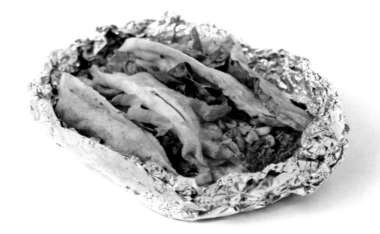

## BELLY BAD

S/C Value = 9/4

Say "adios" to a slender waist with this flour-heavy fixture.

# Tacos with Corn Tortillas

Hola, deliciousness . . . glad you could make it! This tasty, south-of-the-border celebration is full of flavor. How to order: "I'll have corn tacos with carnitas, salsa, sour cream, cheese, guacamole, and lettuce."

## BELLY GOOD

S/C Value = 5/2

# DENNY'S

## Heartland Scramble

## BELLY BAD

S/C Value = 15/6

No amount of fancy footwork will help you scramble out of this breakfast blitz. Remember, 15/6™ is the S/C Value that represents your entire day, not one meal!

# Ultimate Omelette with Side of Hash Browns

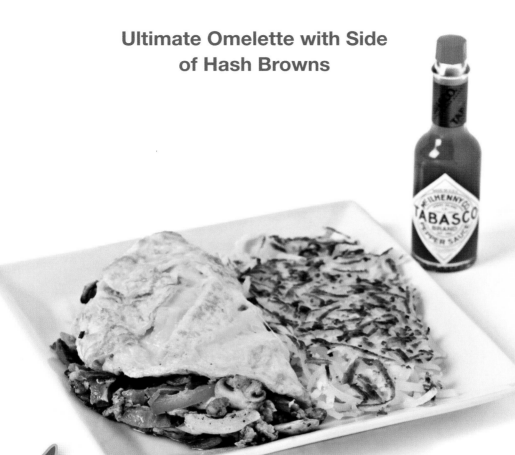

What better way to start your day than with hash browns hot off the griddle, and mushrooms and peppers folded into a savory blanket of eggs? If you're on the go early, this is the ultimate wake-up call.

## BELLY GOOD

S/C Value = 5/2

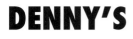

# DENNY'S

## Smoked Chicken Melt

## BELLY BAD

S/C Value = 11/4

This diner delicacy is all smoke and mirrors. Before you're enticed by the words *chicken* and *melt*, pull back the curtain to expose the S/C Value.

# Club Sandwich

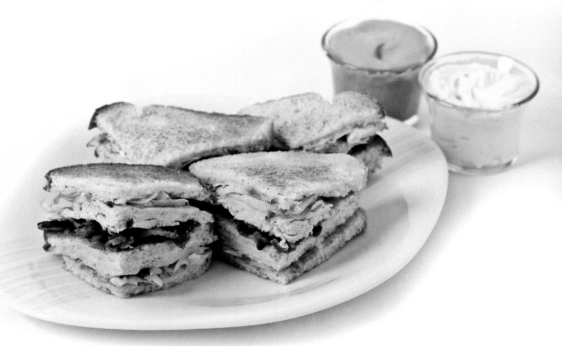

Do you want super-tasty foods and a smaller waistline? Join the club! Order four corners of fresh turkey, crispy bacon, lettuce, mayo, and mustard. How to order: "No tomatoes, please."

## BELLY GOOD

S/C Value = 5/2

# DiGIORNO

Traditional Crust,
Four-Cheese Pizza

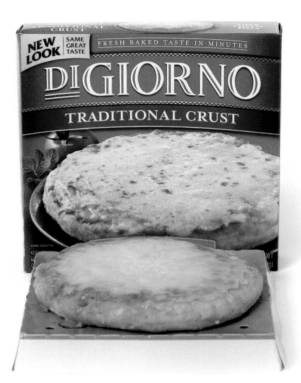

## BELLY BAD

S/C Value = 6/3

As a foodie, I knew pizza needed to be included as a CARB SWAP™. This particular pie didn't make the cut (with 6 grams of sugar per serving, it just misses the mark), but the next page has a saucy number just for you.

# Cheese-Stuffed Crust,
# Four-Cheese Pizza

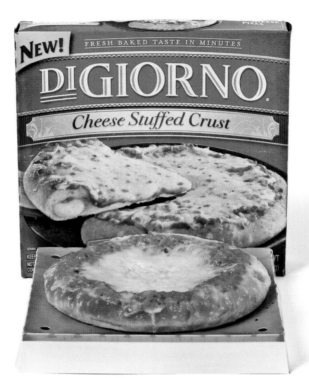

Do I really need to convince you? It's *pizza!* I have a smile on my face just thinking about shoveling a couple slices of heaven into my mouth. The S/C Value is for half of this personal-size pizza.

## BELLY GOOD

S/C Value = 5/2

# DiGIORNO

## Traditional Crust, Supreme Pizza

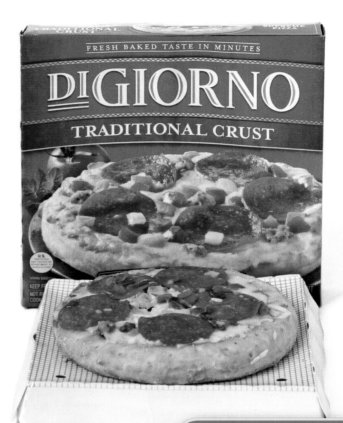

## BELLY BAD

S/C Value = 11/5

Your waistline will be supremely disappointed if you ratchet up insulin levels with this colorful pie.

# Cheese-Stuffed Crust, Pepperoni Pizza

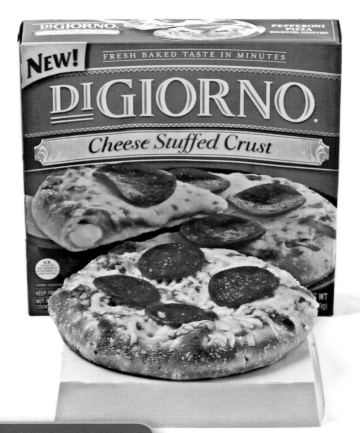

Yep, here's one more piping-hot DiGiorno pie to sink your teeth into. Enjoy half of this personal-size deep dish for a thick layer of mozzarella and a kick of pepperoni. Perfect for two!

## BELLY GOOD

S/C Value = 5/2

## Spaghetti with Meat Sauce

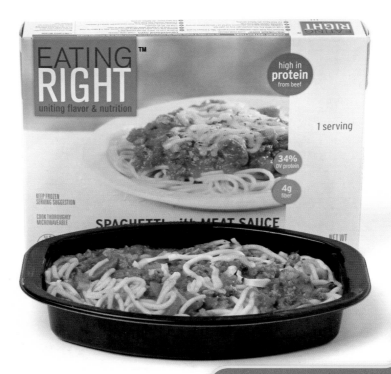

## BELLY BAD

S/C Value = 7/3

> Believe me, there are plenty of places for sugar to hide when the entire dish is covered in marinara.

# Mediterranean-Style Chicken

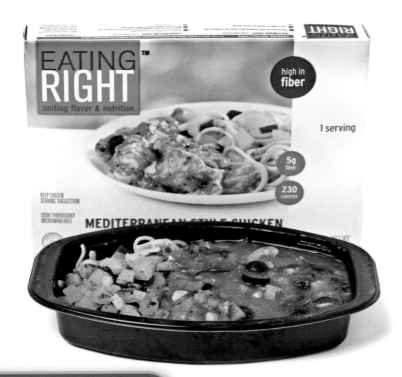

Some say Mediterranean is the way to go, and in this case, I couldn't agree more. Marinara isn't stealing the show this time, and there are plenty of veggies to go around.

## BELLY GOOD

S/C Value = 5/2

## Chicken and
## Vegetable Pot Stickers

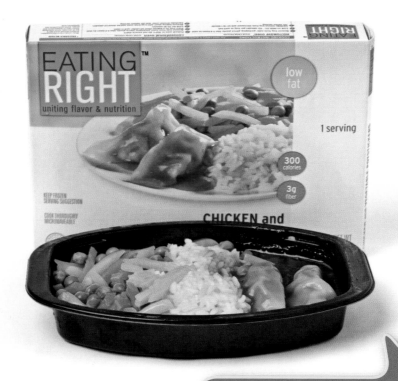

## BELLY BAD

S/C Value = 10/3

Hold up, team . . .
this looks like a sticky
situation for your waistline.
Best to send these
pot stickers packing.

# Chicken with Peanut Sauce

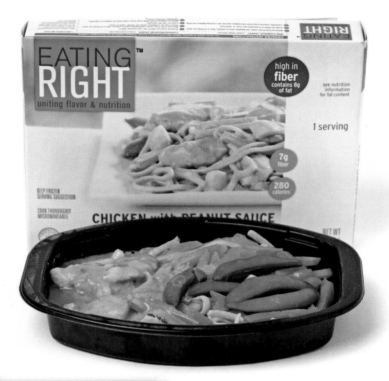

Nothing seedy about this tasty dish. In fact, you'd be nuts to let this plate pass you by! With a rich, flavorful sauce dripping over grilled chicken, eating right never felt so wrong.

## BELLY GOOD

S/C Value = 5/2

## Pineapple Black Bean Chicken

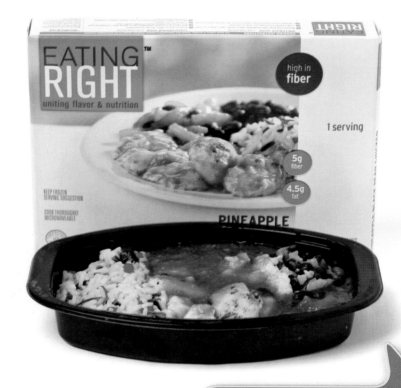

## BELLY BAD

S/C Value = 24/3

Here's another dish that falls into that all-too-familiar category of "Hmm, that sounds healthy . . . " Unfortunately, this pineapple platter is loaded with 24 grams of hidden sugar.

# Fiesta Chicken

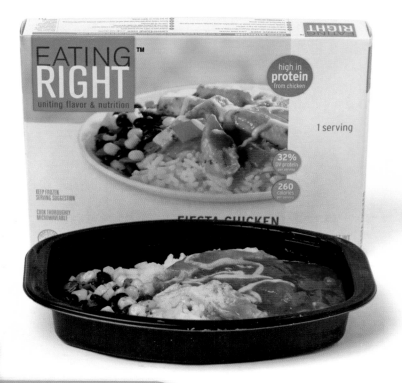

## BELLY GOOD

S/C Value = 2/2

It's time for your
taste buds to party!
Heat up this dish in a hurry
for a flavor celebration.

# EINSTEIN BROS BAGELS

## Cinnamon Raisin Bagel Thin with Reduced-Fat Strawberry Schmear

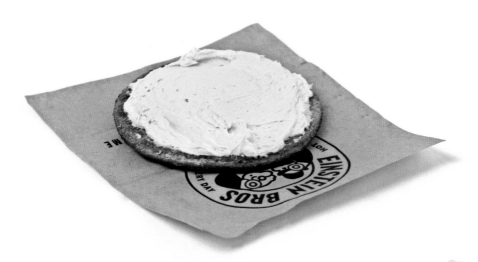

## BELLY BAD

S/C Value = 14/4

Despite how much I love the word *schmear* (it's so much fun to say!) there's a hole in Einstein's "reduced fat" logic: hidden sugar produces insulin, which pushes fat into your cells.

# Nova Lox on an Everything Bagel Thin, with Americano

Have your "schmear" and eat it, too! How to order: "I'll have the Nova Lox on an Everything Thin Bagel with no tomatoes, please." I recommend enjoying this savory sandwich with a patriotic caffeine fix.

## BELLY GOOD

S/C Value = 5/2

# EINSTEIN BROS BAGELS

## Tasty Turkey on an Asiago Cheese Bagel

## BELLY BAD

S/C Value = 9/4

Talk about a "tasty" scandal . . . better read the fine print before you sign your belly away to this sandwich. You're about to get swindled into a high S/C Value.

# Turkey-Breast Deli Sandwich
## on Challah

This scrumptious sandwich is worth betting your belly on. You're about to build your own royal flush of deli flavor. How to order: "Oven-roasted turkey, Swiss cheese, and mustard on challah, please." I'm all in!

## BELLY GOOD

S/C Value = 5/2

# HEALTHY CHOICE

## Café Steamers
## Whiskey Steak

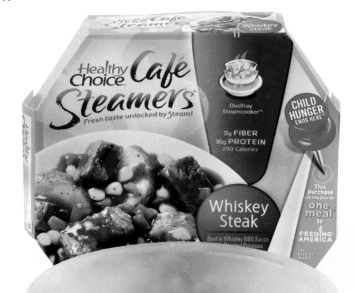

## BELLY BAD

S/C Value = 20/3

This whiskey sauce is the definition of hidden sugar. It actually blows my mind how Healthy Choice managed to fit 20 grams into this meager plate of food.

# Café Steamers
# Roasted Beef Merlot

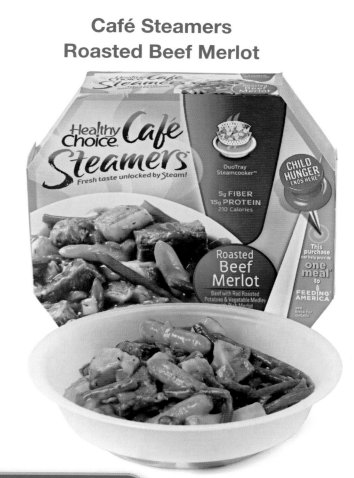

> Merlot always seems to bring class to a meal, and this is no exception. So here's to healthy proteins, fiber, and vitamin A . . . cheers!

## BELLY GOOD

S/C Value = 5/2

# HEALTHY CHOICE

## Café Steamers Sweet Sesame Chicken

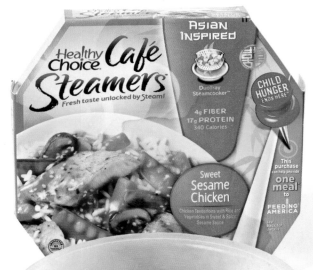

## BELLY BAD

S/C Value = 19/3

This Asian-inspired dish is nothing to write home about . . . unless you want to send a postcard of your expanding waistline.

# Café Steamers Roasted Chicken Fresca

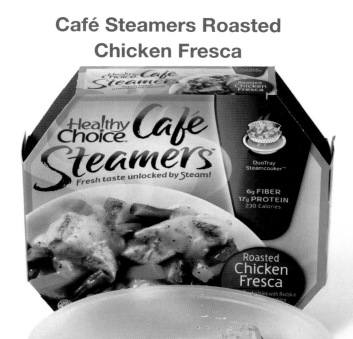

No need for intercontinental travel to enjoy this delicious, "just like Mom used to make" chicken dish. Just visit your local supermarket and head straight to the freezer.

## BELLY GOOD

S/C Value = 3/2

# HEALTHY CHOICE

## Café Steamers
## Beef Teriyaki

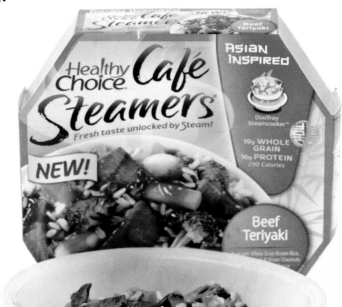

## BELLY BAD

S/C Value = 16/3

You can claim this meal is healthy till the cows come home, but it won't change the fact that this meal packs one heifer of an S/C Value.

# Café Steamers Grilled Basil Chicken

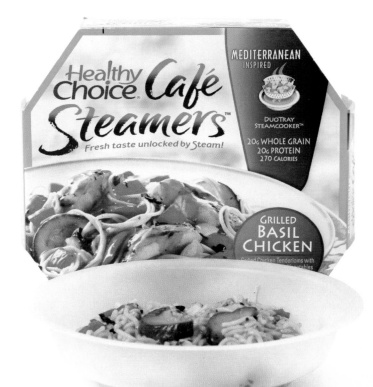

Dear Grilled Basil Chicken, there's so much I want to say. I mean, you really are just a super-tasty pasta dish that has it all: healthy protein, yummy pasta, and a low sugar value. In short, you rock!

## BELLY GOOD

S/C Value = 4/2

## Fresh-Fruit Crepe with Blueberry Compote

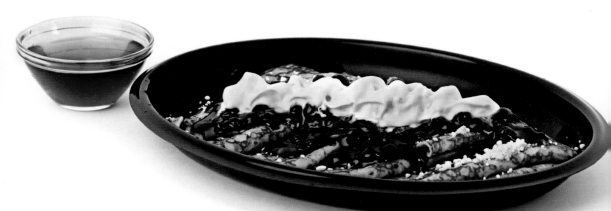

## BELLY BAD

S/C Value = 44/4

Yes, it sounds exotic—and, yes, blueberries tug at your heartstrings. But this sexy selection will only betray your belly with 3 days' worth of sugar in the morning. Tell this dish to pack its bags.

# Bacon Temptation
## Omelette

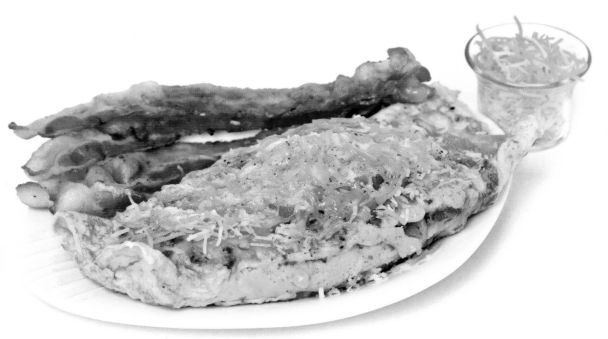

Here's your chance to give in to temptation. Surrender to your palate's passion with this flavor fest. Indulge in crispy bacon and melted cheese folded together in a fried egg. You'll be glad you did.

## BELLY GOOD

S/C Value = 5/1

## Crispy Chicken Salad

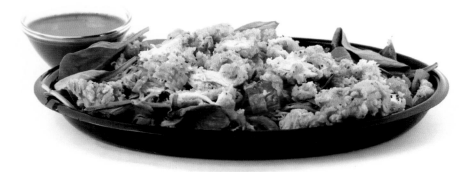

## BELLY BAD

S/C Value = 15/4

I get it: you see spinach and it triggers something healthy in your subconscious. But this plate of hidden sugar is only masquerading as Belly Good. Ignore the clever disguise.

# Grilled Chicken Salad and Chicken Tortilla Soup

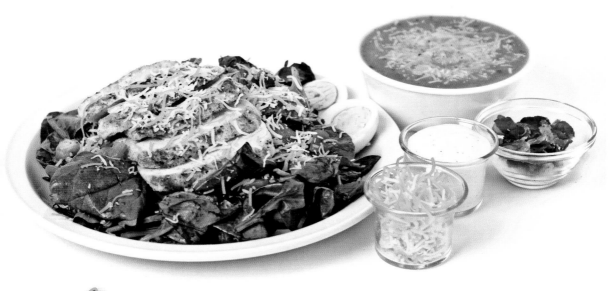

Talk about more flavor and less belly! How to customize your order: "I'll have spinach salad with grilled chicken, crumbled bacon, Caesar dressing, cheese, and a cup of chicken tortilla soup."

## BELLY GOOD

S/C Value = 3/2

# JACK IN THE BOX

## Ultimate
## Breakfast Sandwich

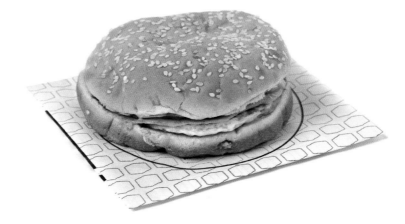

## BELLY BAD

S/C Value = 6/3

First of all, who puts a breakfast sandwich on a sesame-seed bun? That's not "ultimate," that's just silly. Second, it's a problem to consume nearly half your daily sugar value in one meal.

# Supreme Croissant, and Coffee with Cream

Ah, the French are at it again. This time, their flaky roll inspires a tasty, European-style swap. This delicious sandwich boasts a fried egg, layered ham, two types of cheese, and crispy bacon.

## BELLY GOOD

S/C Value = 4/2

# JACK IN THE BOX

## Mini Sirloin Burgers

## BELLY BAD

S/C Value = 19/4

> This miniature meal is like cuddling with a baby tiger: adorable, playful . . . and a natural-born killer. There's nothing safe (or mini!) about the impact this S/C Value will have on your waistline.

# Sourdough Steak Melt

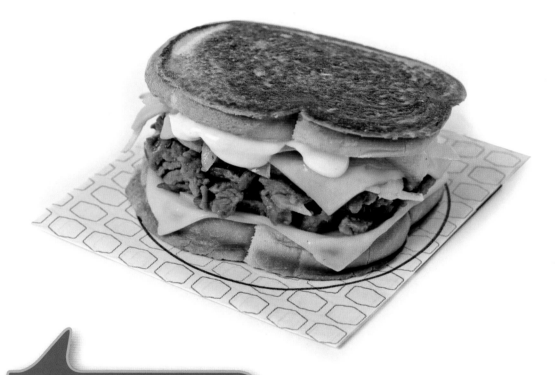

## BELLY GOOD

S/C Value = 5/2

## Homestyle-Ranch Chicken Club

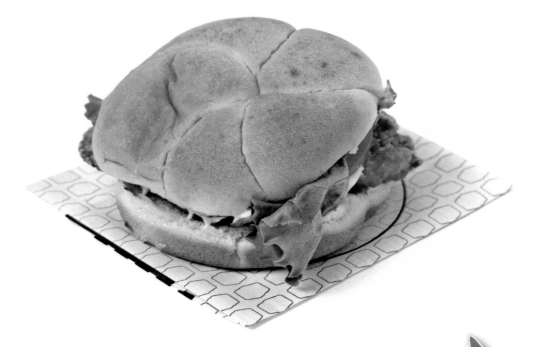

## BELLY BAD

S/C Value = 8/4

> The heartwarming title may promise homegrown flavor, but you might want to take a look at the S/C Value before you kick back on the porch swing.

# Sourdough
# Grilled-Chicken Club

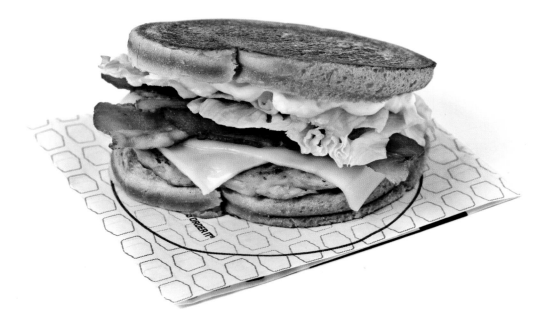

Now this is thinking outside the box: a fresh, flavorful club that's Belly Fat Cure™ approved. How to order: "No tomatoes, please."

## BELLY GOOD

S/C Value = 5/2

# JACK IN THE BOX

## Grilled Chicken Salad

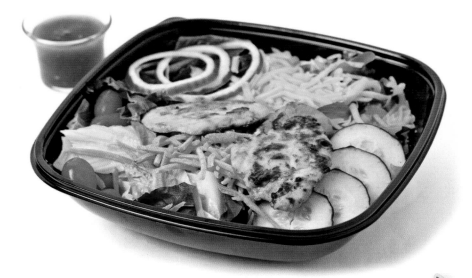

## BELLY BAD

S/C Value = 10/2

Careful again of the sneaky, "low-fat" phrasing in that balsamic vinaigrette. Makes me wonder if they think I don't know jack . . . at 10 sugar grams total, I promise we can get a better salad with more flavor.

# Chicken Club Salad and Mozzarella Cheese Sticks

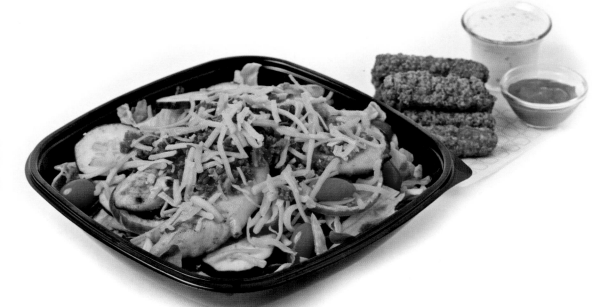

"Plenty of fresh greens, veggies, layered with delicious cheese and bacon, blah blah blah . . . does that say mozzarella cheese sticks?" Absolutely! And you're not the only one excited about it!

## BELLY GOOD

S/C Value = 5/2

## Sweet & Sour Chicken

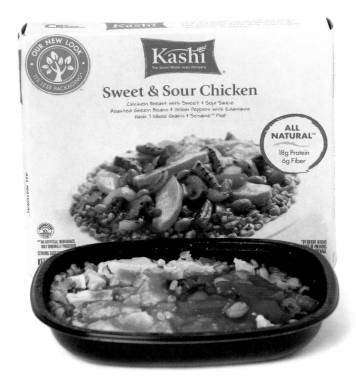

## BELLY BAD

### S/C Value = 25/3

All the "sweet" in this Chinese staple makes it "sour" for your waistline. There's no shame in chickening out when you consider the S/C Value of this take-out classic.

# Chicken Pasta Pomodoro

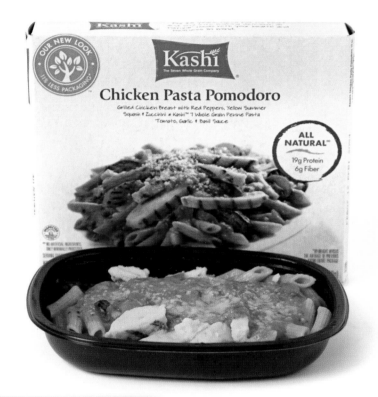

If your heart skips a beat when you hear "pasta," then you and I have something in common! This succulent pasta dish is flavored with a scrumptious, low-sugar tomato sauce with garlic and basil.

## BELLY GOOD

S/C Value = 5/2

# KASHI

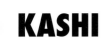

## Mayan Harvest Bake

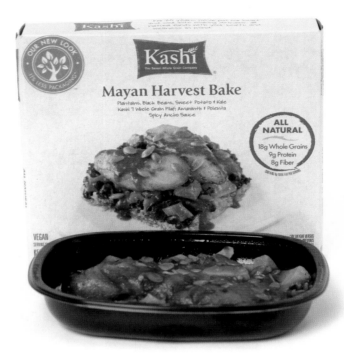

## BELLY BAD

**S/C Value = 19/3**

> You'd think with all their infamous predictions, the Mayans could've foreseen a high sugar count in this dish. I predict your waistline will definitely grow after you eat this dish.

# Pesto Pasta Primavera

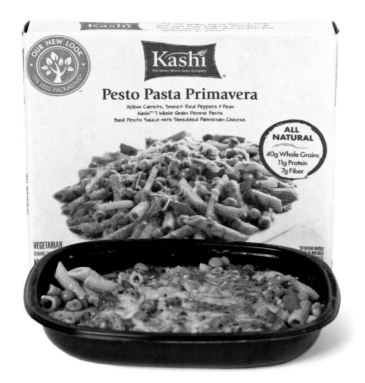

This Belly Good meal is brought to you by "taste" and the letter "P." This prima, pasta-licious plate is perfect for your pancreas.

## BELLY GOOD

S/C Value = 4/2

## Honey BBQ Sandwich

## BELLY BAD

S/C Value = 21/3

"Honey, can you pass the high S/C Value?" Barbeque sauce is tough to keep out of the Belly Bad club. This meal seems to want a lifetime membership.

# Ultimate Cheese KFC Snacker

With a meal this healthy, double dipping is 100 percent permitted. My recommendation? Go to town on this cheesy, tasty wonder.

## BELLY GOOD

S/C Value = 5/2

# Chicken Pot Pie

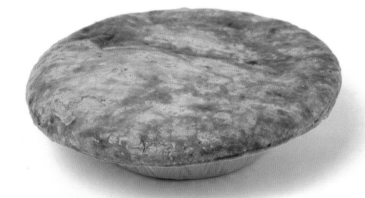

## BELLY BAD

S/C Value = 7/4

This meal is heavy on the "pie" and light on the "chicken." I'd rather get this pie in the face than actually eat it. At least then we could laugh about it!

# Grilled 3-Piece Meal with Green Beans, Mashed Potatoes with Gravy, and 3" Corn on the Cob

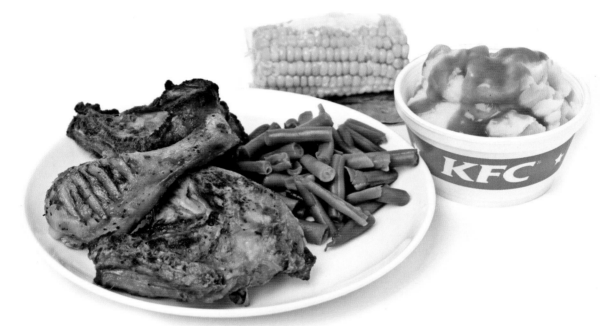

This meal is the definition of "finger-lickin' good"! Each piece of grilled chicken is 0/0, so dig in! I recommend pairing your protein with green beans, mashed potatoes with gravy, and a 3" piece of corn on the cob.

## BELLY GOOD

S/C Value = 4/2

# 3 Fiery Buffalo Wings
# with Cole Slaw and Home-Style Biscuit

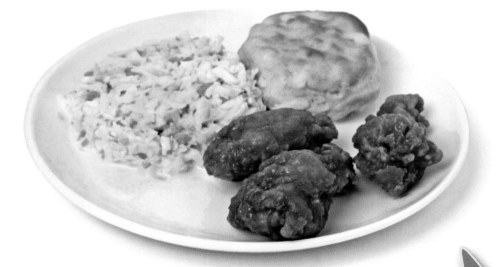

## BELLY BAD

### S/C Value = 28/4

This spicy mix is a real S/C firecracker. But it's not the Buffalo sauce that will get you in trouble— it's the mound of cole slaw.

# 3 Original Recipe Wings with Green Beans and Home-Style Biscuit

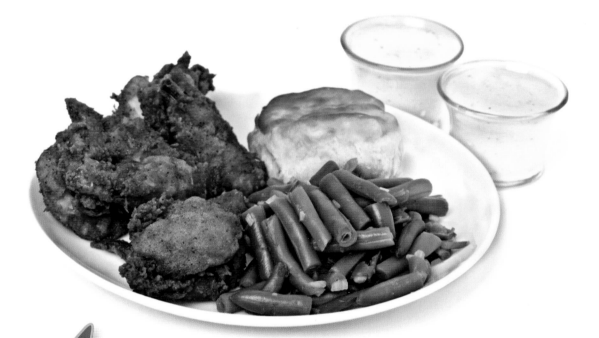

I wish I had something original to say about all this food . . . honestly, it's just plain good! For those of you not sold on the biscuit alone, I've added tasty wings and buttermilk ranch dressing.

## BELLY GOOD

S/C Value = 5/2

## Grilled Chicken & Penne Pasta

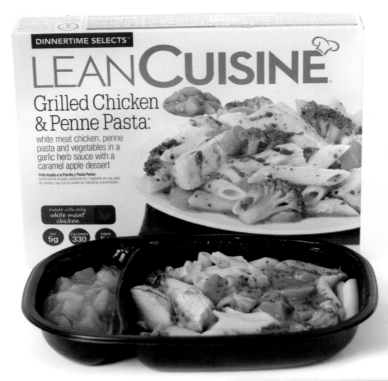

## BELLY BAD

S/C Value = 24/3

The name's Sugar . . . Hidden Sugar. Someone less savvy than you might consider this meal healthy. But you're a special agent trained to identify sugar, and this threat has been neutralized.

# Lemon Pepper Fish

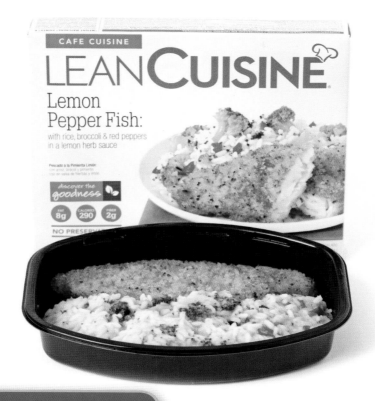

Lean Cuisine is about to hook you up with the Catch of the Day! Enjoy scrumptious fish with fresh lemon flavor and a pop of pepper.

## BELLY GOOD

S/C Value = 4/2

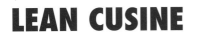
## Beef and Broccoli

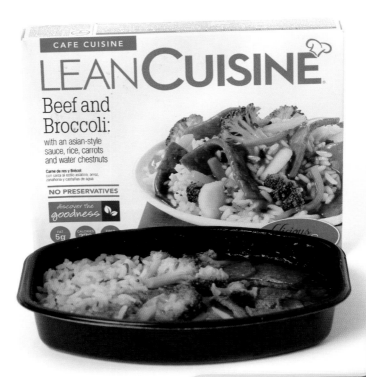

## BELLY BAD

S/C Value = 9/3

Unbelievable, a beef and broccoli fail. And this is such an easy one to get right . . . I'm actually devastated by this one. I love mixing up my meat and veggies, but sadly this mash-up misses the mark.

# Salisbury Steak
# with Macaroni and Cheese

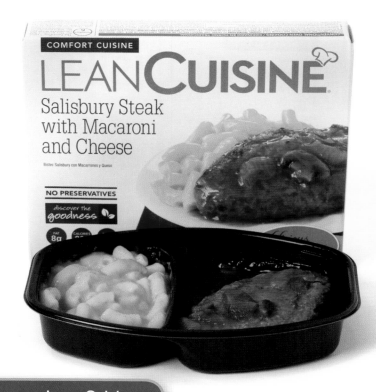

I'm pretty sure Lean Cuisine has some kind of superpower. Just when it seemed all hope was lost, they swooped in with this bodacious combo to save the day!

## BELLY GOOD

S/C Value = 3/2

# LEAN CUISINE

## Roasted Turkey Breast

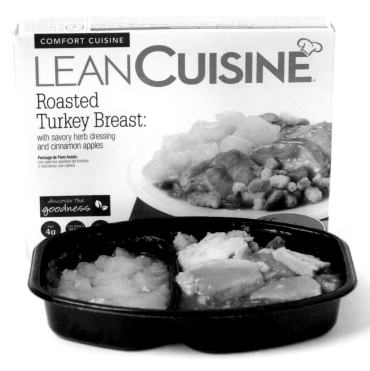

## BELLY BAD

S/C Value = 27/3

Anyone who truly wants to be lean should steer clear of this meal. It doesn't take a keen eye to realize the real culprit here: cinnamon apples. This sugary entrée is off-limits.

# Salmon with Basil

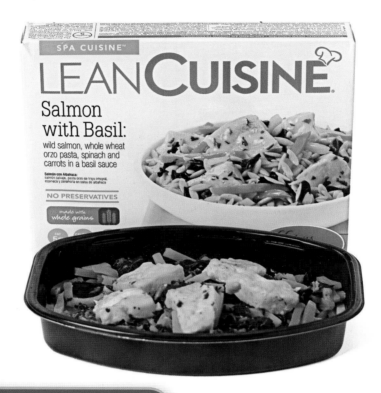

Lean Cuisine is making a statement: salmon is the new turkey. With ingredients this delicious, there's nothing fishy about this choice.

## BELLY GOOD

S/C Value = 2/2

# LEAN CUISINE

## Sweet & Spicy Ginger Chicken

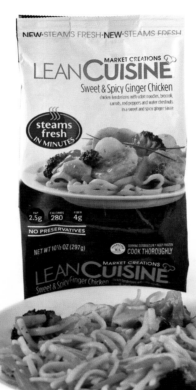

## BELLY BAD

S/C Value = 12/3

This meal is like the "Where's Waldo?" of ginger chicken. It would be easier to find the chicken strips in this skimpy selection if they were wearing red and white caps. Oh, and it has a poor S/C Value to boot.

# Lemon Garlic Shrimp

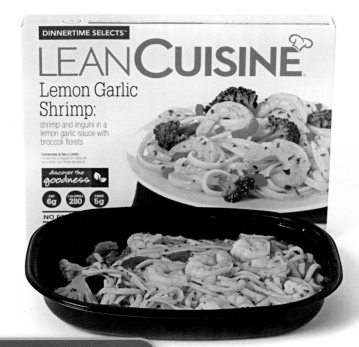

Ooh la la! A sultry dish with flavor in all the right places. Go ahead, take a closer look: curvaceous shrimp dripping with lemon flavor and a kick of garlic. No need to ask, I'll give you its digits: 3/2.

## BELLY GOOD

S/C Value = 3/2

# LEAN POCKETS

## Cheeseburger

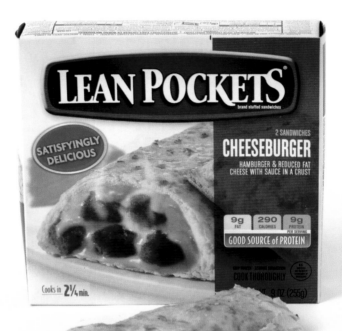

## BELLY BAD

S/C Value = 9/3

Maybe this is the hidden sugar talking, but I suppose it was only a matter of time before a burger was packaged up in pocket form. Innovative? Sure. But the numbers aren't flattering at all.

# Grilled Chicken Jalapeño Cheddar Pretzel Bread

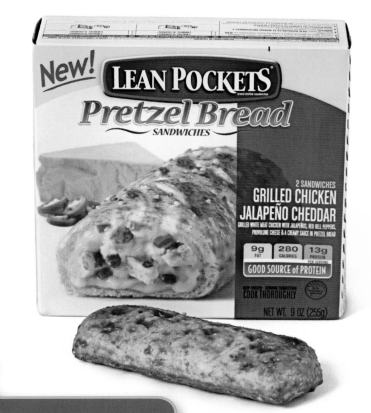

Now here's a pocket with enough personality to keep you curious. This zippy combo brings together grilled chicken, melted cheddar, and spicy jalapeño all wrapped up (guilt-free) in a convenient, flaky shell.

## BELLY GOOD

S/C Value = 2/2

# LONG JOHN SILVER'S

## Breaded Clam Strips with Corn Cobbette

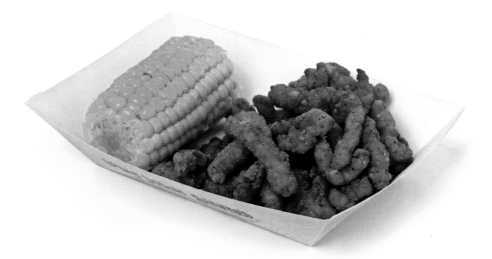

## BELLY BAD

S/C Value = 7/3

My waistline is starting to clam up. Truthfully, I have no idea how Captain Silver finagles clams into strips—and quite frankly, I don't want to know! Regardless, the S/C Value of this dish is just plain fishy.

# 6-Piece Battered Shrimp with 2 Hush Puppies

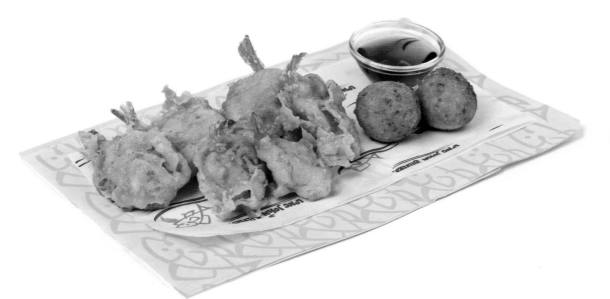

Show me the hush puppies! As incredible as this might seem, those luscious lumps in all their deep-fried glory plus six pieces of succulent, battered shrimp equals one tasty Belly Good meal.

## BELLY GOOD

S/C Value = 2/2

# LONG JOHN SILVER'S

## Freshside Grille Shrimp Scampi and Cole Slaw

## BELLY BAD

S/C Value = 19/2

> Best to scamper away from this saucy concoction before your waistline gets grilled. Not even veggies can save you from a cole-slaw-heavy, hidden sugar count that's far from shrimpy.

# Freshside Grille Salmon Entrée with Lobster Bites

I'm about to win over your taste buds with a savory, seaside delight. Get ready for grilled salmon, an array of veggies, and infamous morsels of supernatural flavor: lobster bites. My work here is done.

## BELLY GOOD

S/C Value = 4/2

# MARIE CALLENDER'S

## Sweet & Sour Chicken

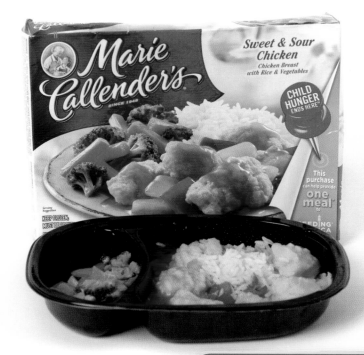

## BELLY BAD

S/C Value = 35/5

> Your sweet dream of a slender waistline is about to turn sour. The syrupy sauce drowning these breaded morsels is full of hidden sugar.

# Chunky Chicken & Noodles

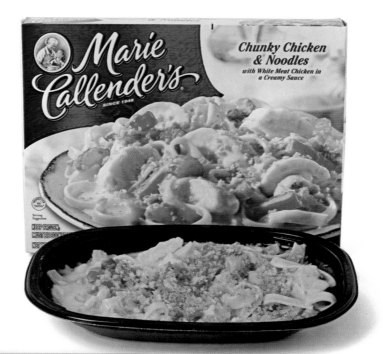

Even if the word *chunky* doesn't exactly court your senses, I promise that this plentiful plate will meet your every desire. Marie brings this kitchen classic to life with nifty noodles and thick bites of fresh chicken.

## BELLY GOOD

S/C Value = 2/2

# MARIE CALLENDER'S

## Chicken Santa Fe

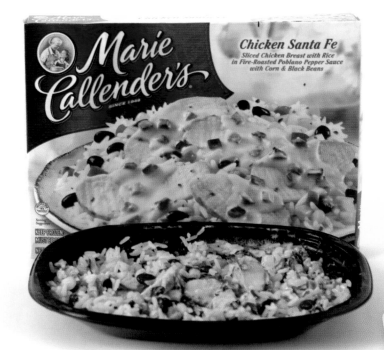

## BELLY BAD

S/C Value = 6/3

Southwestern flavor is among my favorites, but as your coach, I have to draw the line. The S/C Value may not be off the charts, but it's certainly enough to get you off track.

# Herb Roasted Chicken

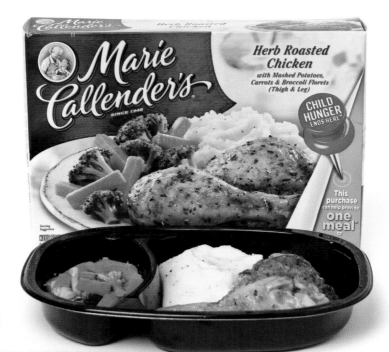

How about this herb-o-rific entrée? Savory, seasoned chicken with a super-duper S/C Value . . . it's a CARB SWAP™ success!

## BELLY GOOD

S/C Value = 3/2

# MARIE CALLENDER'S

## Sesame Chicken

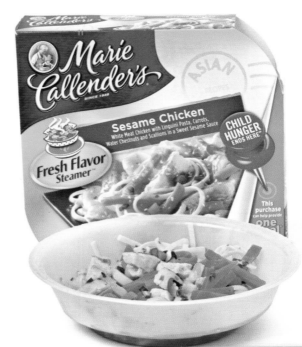

## BELLY BAD

S/C Value = 22/3

Open sesame! Wait, I mean "close"—close sesame! This edible odyssey is not one you want your belly to embark on. The only treasure in this cave of wonders is hidden sugar. Keep it to yourself, Ali Baba!

# Chicken Fajita Bowl

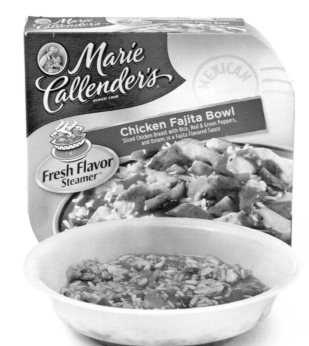

As the old saying goes, "Everything tastes better in a bowl." Okay, maybe that's not an actual saying, but in this case it should be: grilled chicken, bell peppers, and onions in a tasty fajita sauce. Delicioso!

## BELLY GOOD

S/C Value = 4/2

# MARIE CALLENDER'S

## Chicken Teriyaki

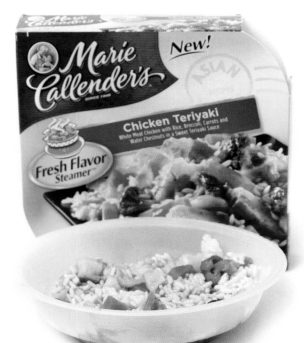

## BELLY BAD

S/C Value = 14/3

This sugar-heavy dish is like playing chicken with your waistline. In Lady Callender's defense, it *is* difficult to deliver a tasty, low-sugar teriyaki dish. Nonetheless, this tropical marinade is off-limits.

# Chicken Stir-Fry with Vegetables

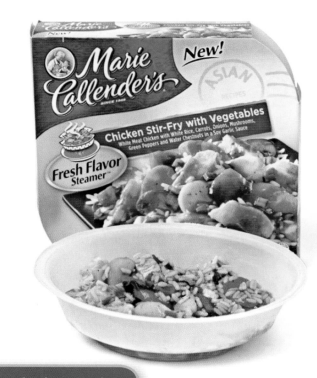

I'm not sure who invented stir-fry, but I would like to shake their hand. Maybe give 'em a hug. Marie definitely gets another one right, so reach for your chopsticks and dive into deliciousness!

## BELLY GOOD

S/C Value = 4/2

# McDONALD'S

## Sausage, Egg & Cheese McGriddle

## BELLY BAD

S/C Value = 15/3

I guess it's not really hidden sugar if you can actually see the maple crystals imbedded in the bun. It shouldn't surprise you that this breakfast gem has a full day's worth of sugar.

# Egg McMuffin

For those of you who love the familiar aroma of this McDonald's favorite first thing in the morning, take heart: this traditional breakfast sandwich is both delicious *and* Belly Fat Cure™ approved!

## BELLY GOOD

S/C Value = 3/2

# McDONALD'S

## Hotcakes with Syrup

## BELLY BAD

S/C Value = 46/6

The fast-food giant truly lives up to its old "super-size" reputation with this stack of pure sugar. With 3 days' worth of hidden sugar and 6 servings of carbs, this meal is literally a belly-fat *accelerator.*

# Bacon, Egg & Cheese Biscuit

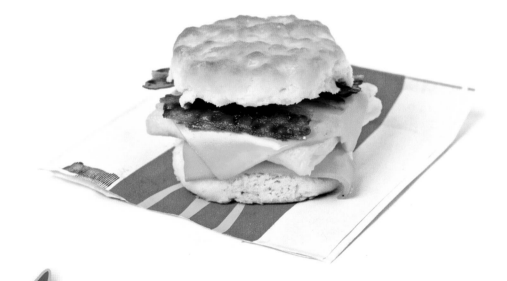

This is the bright, birds-chirping, sun-rising-on-the-horizon day to the pancake's night: crispy bacon, fresh egg, and melted American cheese layered on a buttery biscuit. The S/C Value and taste both hit the spot.

## BELLY GOOD

S/C Value = 3/2

# McDONALD'S

## 4-Piece Chicken McNuggets with Honey-Mustard Sauce

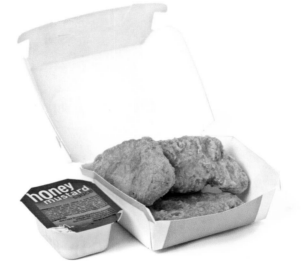

## BELLY BAD

S/C Value = 8/2

It's definitely hit or miss under the golden arches. At 8 grams of sugar, this is a miss. Also, here's a nugget of wisdom for you: honey mustard is full of hidden sugar, so swap this meal!

# 3 Chicken Selects Premium Breast Strips with Spicy Buffalo Sauce

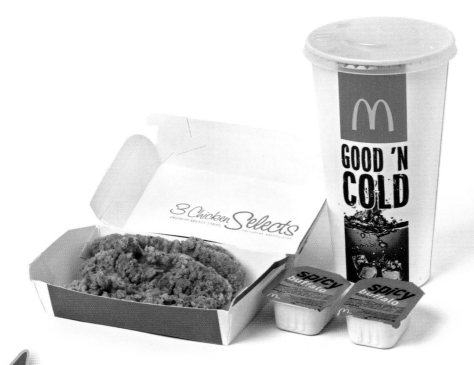

All swaps are Coach Jorge approved, but this is actually a personal favorite of mine. Crunchy, flavorful strips of all-white meat dipped in zippy Buffalo sauce . . . I really *am* loving it!

## BELLY GOOD

S/C Value = 0/2

**Big Mac**

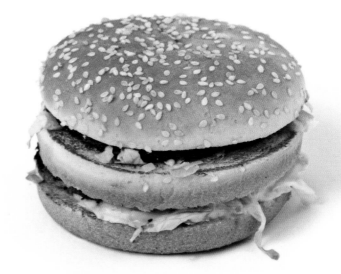

## BELLY BAD

S/C Value = 9/3

That's right, not even McDonald's trademark burger is safe from my mission to cure belly fat! It would take a bold, misguided Mickey D's junkie to come to the defense of this S/C Value.

# McChicken Sandwich

Here's a McHealthier choice to help you drop McBelly Fat. When you need a tasty sandwich on the go, this one delivers delicious fried chicken topped with cheese, lettuce, and mayo on a warm bun.

## BELLY GOOD

S/C Value = 5/2

# McDONALD'S

## Premium Grilled Chicken Classic Sandwich

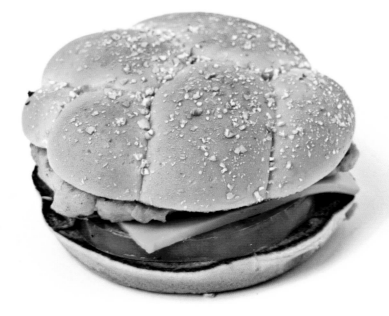

## BELLY BAD

S/C Value = 11/3

Despite its all-American charm, this meal packs some pretty miserable statistics. Avoid a classic error by leaving this sandwich on the warming tray.

# Filet-O-Fish

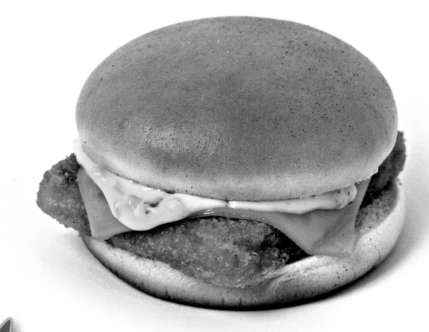

Here's a McDonald's classic that needs no introduction. But I'll give it one anyway: "Aaaand now, hailing from the Atlantic (probably), battered, fried, and ready for action, it's . . . Filet-O-Fish!"

## BELLY GOOD

S/C Value = 5/2

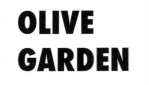

# OLIVE GARDEN

## Calamari with Marinara Sauce and Berry Sangria

**BELLY BAD**

S/C Value = 36/3

> I know that "berry sangria" sounds pleasant, but I promise it's packed with hidden sugar. The second red flag in this entrée is "marinara" . . . same deal.

# Stuffed Mushrooms
# and Red Wine

Mmm . . . I see cheese-stuffed mushrooms and I'm all in. This flavorful meal will keep you satisfied long after the wine wears off.

## BELLY GOOD

S/C Value = 3/2

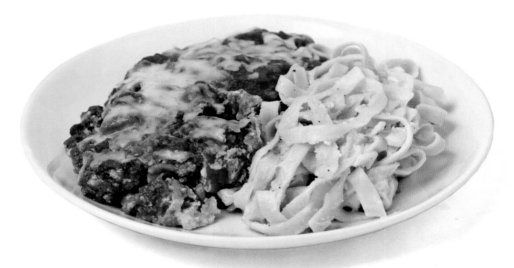

## BELLY BAD

**S/C Value = 12/5**

Hello, my name is Jorge, and I'll be your tour guide. As a reminder, please keep all forks inside the vehicle. If you take a look down at your plate, you'll see nearly a full day's worth of carbs in one meal. . . .

# Stuffed Chicken Marsala

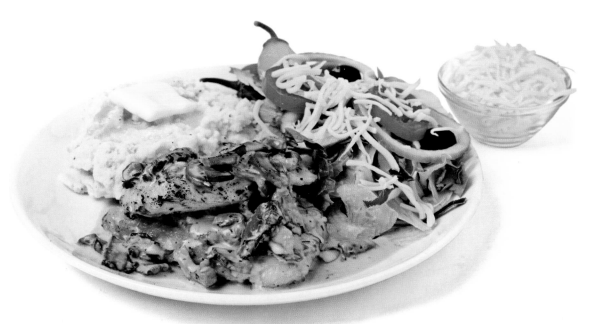

This flavorful selection is a perfect 10, so close your eyes and breathe in the aroma of guilt-free flavor. Savor this delicious dish for a slender waistline when you're out.

## BELLY GOOD

S/C Value = 3/2

# OLIVE GARDEN

## Venetian Apricot Chicken

## BELLY BAD

S/C Value = 14/2

So many seductive words in one place . . . I guess that's just Italy for you. Still, know when you read that exotic name that the true destination is your waistline.

# Grilled Chicken Spiedini

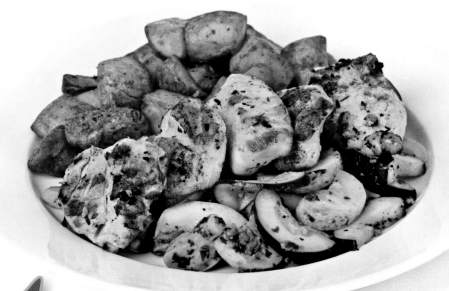

**BELLY GOOD**

S/C Value = 3/2

A truly splendid selection for your shrinking waistline. Honestly, what's not to love? Magnifico!

# OLIVE GARDEN

## Eggplant Parmigiana

## BELLY BAD

S/C Value = 15/5

The only type of planting you'll be doing after consuming this carbo-loaded dish is the one involving your behind on the couch!

# Parmesan-Crusted Bistecca

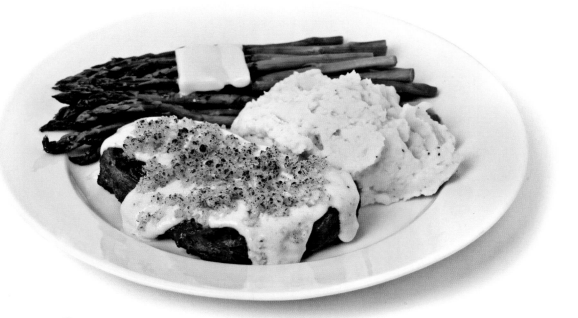

Now here's a dish I can really sink my teeth into: a potent combo featuring juicy steak and fresh asparagus. Where's the nearest Olive Garden?

## BELLY GOOD

S/C Value = 3/2

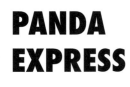

## PANDA EXPRESS

**Beijing Beef**

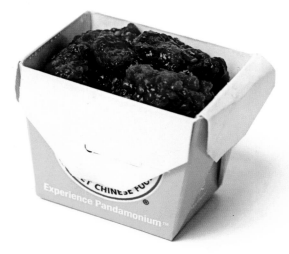

## BELLY BAD

S/C Value = 23/3

Break open your fortune cookie and see if it says this: "Give hidden sugar a chance this week. Your belly-growing plans will be successful." Let me enlighten you to the unlucky numbers of its S/C Value: 23/3.

# Broccoli Beef, Mixed Veggies, and Fried Rice

This delicious meal looks like it could satisfy an actual Panda. How to order: "I'll have a two-entrée plate with Mixed Veggies and Broccoli Beef, and just a quarter serving of rice."

## BELLY GOOD

S/C Value = 5/2

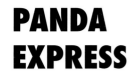

## Golden Treasure Shrimp

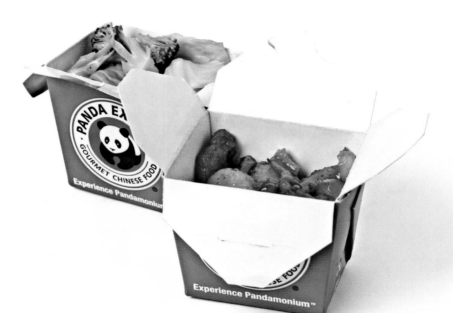

## BELLY BAD

S/C Value = 19/3

This golden treasure will expand your belly, not your bank account. There are plenty of Belly Good shrimp dishes in this book (including a tasty swap on the next page), so please don't let this one break your heart.

# Crispy Shrimp with Mixed Veggies

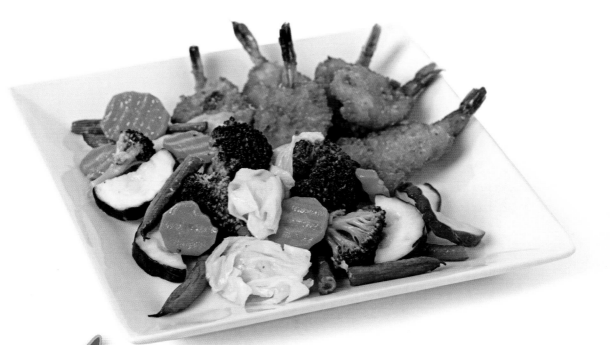

Jackpot! Enjoy tasty shrimp and a flatter belly. How to order: "I'll have a two-entrée plate (no rice or chow mein, please) with Crispy Shrimp and Mixed Veggies."

## BELLY GOOD

S/C Value = 4/2

# PANDA EXPRESS

## Chicken Egg Roll with Mandarin Sauce, and 3 Chicken Pot Stickers

**POTSTICKER SAUCE**

PANDA EXPRESS
GOURMET CHINESE FOOD

## BELLY BAD

S/C Value = 22/3

If you're starting to think that Panda could be man or woman's new best friend, you might want to reconsider. This wild animal has some S/C Values that are difficult to tame.

# Mushroom Chicken and 2 Spring Rolls

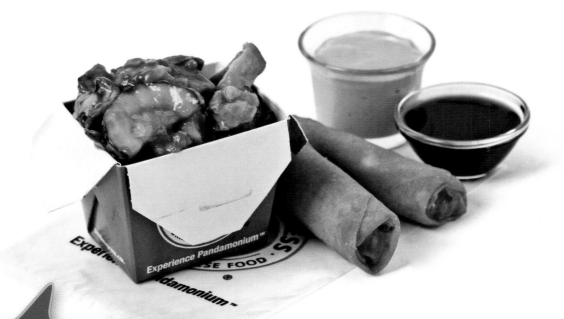

"You had me at 'spring rolls.'" Right?! But this flavor romance is far from over. Your chopsticks have a savory rendezvous planned with grilled veggies and tempting chicken morsels dripping with delicious sauce.

## BELLY GOOD

S/C Value = 5/2

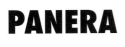

## Tuna Salad Sandwich
## on Honey Wheat Bread

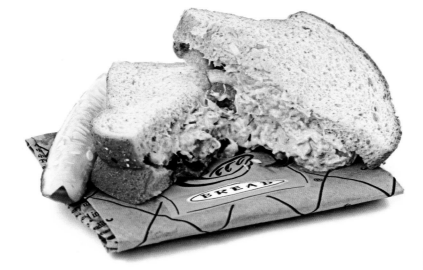

### BELLY BAD

S/C Value = 12/4

> As a foodie, the word *bread* always excites my senses. Because of that, I need to choose my carbs wisely. This one is a no-go, but trust me, there's plenty of taste on the horizon.

# Half Asiago Roast Beef Sandwich and Half a Classic Salad

As your carb guru, I invite you to meditate on savory roast beef on cheese-infused bread. How to order: "I'll have the 'You Pick Two,' with half an Asiago Roast Beef Sandwich and half a Classic Salad with Greek dressing."

## BELLY GOOD

S/C Value = 4/2

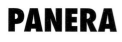

## Fuji Apple
## Chicken Salad

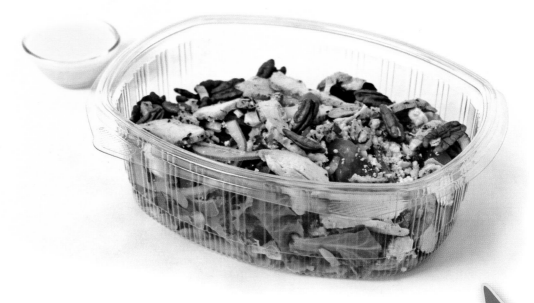

## BELLY BAD

S/C Value = 31/3

This edible wonder is closer to a candy apple than a salad. Tell Johnny Appleseed to take his two days of hidden sugar and hit the road.

# Grilled Chicken
# Caesar Salad

In the Roman Empire, Julius Caesar considered this the salad of the gods . . . probably. No, I can't actually back that up historically, but I think that this Mount Olympus of fresh greens is divine!

## BELLY GOOD

S/C Value = 3/2

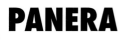

# PANERA

## Sausage, Egg & Cheese on French Toast Bagel

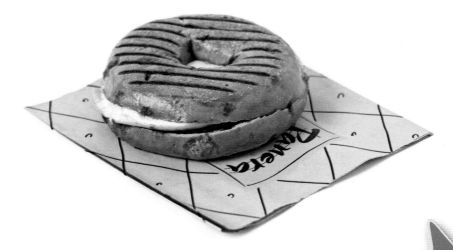

## BELLY BAD

S/C Value = 15/4

> Despite its French-inspired origins, there's not a whole lot of romance in this breakfast sandwich. And that S/C Value—yikes. Definitely a deal-breaker.

# Breakfast Power Sandwich and Coffee with Cream

Here's an aptly titled breakfast sandwich with plenty of tasty, nutritional force behind it. Empower yourself with crispy bacon and smoked ham for an explosive start to your day.

## BELLY GOOD

S/C Value = 2/2

# POPEYES

## Chicken Po' Boy

## BELLY BAD

S/C Value = 10/2

This po' boy is a po' choice for your po' belly. Stuffing fried chicken in a floury bun packed with hidden sugar doesn't exactly make for a good time. Best to leave the po' boy alone.

# 3 Piece Louisiana Tenders with Biscuit

Seasoned strips of fried chicken with ranch dipping sauce and a melt-in-your-mouth biscuit will satisfy your senses and your sensibility with an S/C Value with true Southern hospitality.

## BELLY GOOD

S/C Value = 2/2

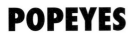
# POPEYES

## 6 Piece Chicken Nuggets
## with Cole Slaw

## BELLY BAD

S/C Value = 15/2

This sloppy side to your nuggets will not be slaw-ving your belly-fat problem. As unassuming as that cup o' cabbage and carrot slivers might seem, it's actually dripping with an entire day's worth of sugar.

# 6 Piece Chicken Nuggets
## with Chicken & Sausage Jambalaya

That isn't just your stomach growling . . . it's the sound of your deepest cravings celebrating. Yes, this soulful selection of crispy chicken with ranch and zesty jambalaya will have your taste buds doing a two-step.

## BELLY GOOD

S/C Value = 3/2

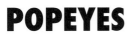

# POPEYES

## Red Beans & Rice
## with Corn on the Cob

## BELLY BAD

S/C Value = 9/4

This unholy roller is ready to knock you off the straight and narrow. We don't need no trouble round these parts, cowboy . . . take your heaping pile of hidden sugar and *get*.

# 3 Pieces of Chicken with Mashed Potatoes and Gravy

Embrace your Southern roots and wash those blues away with comfort food at its finest! Here's the gospel truth, y'all: zero sugar, and only 2 servings of carbs. Can I get an "Amen"?!

## BELLY GOOD

S/C Value = 0/2

# QUIZNOS

## Roadhouse Steak Flatbread Sammie with Small Tomato Basil Soup

## BELLY BAD

S/C Value = 17/3

This soup 'n' Sammie is a real whammy for your waistline. The soup alone puts your sugar count above your limit for one meal.

# Alpine Chicken Flatbread Sammie with Small Broccoli Cheese Soup

> If someone dressed as this Sammie were spinning a Quiznos sign on the side of the road, I would immediately pull over and give him a running high five. How to order: "No dressing, please."

## BELLY GOOD

S/C Value = 5/2

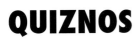

# QUIZNOS

## Raspberry Chipotle Chicken Salad with Small Chili

## BELLY BAD

S/C Value = 25/3

C'mon, Quiznos, this ain't my first rodeo! You can't trick me into thinking that something is healthy by putting fruit in the title. I know my hidden sugar. Ha, *real* raspberries are *low* in sugar. . . good try, though.

# Chicken Taco Salad with Large Chicken Noodle Soup

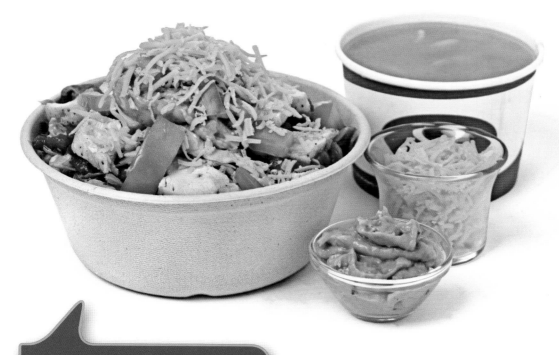

Talk about a flavorful family classic with a side of fiesta. It's like Mom is comforting you with hot chicken noodle soup and throwing you a party at the same time.

## BELLY GOOD

S/C Value = 5/2

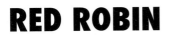

# RED ROBIN

## Jumbo Shrimp and Coleslaw

## BELLY BAD

S/C Value = 27/5

Arr, me mateys, prepare your waistline to walk the plank! Talk about trouble on the high seas: this meal rocks the boat with 27 grams of sugar and 5 servings of carbs . . . and that's without fries!

# Arctic Cod with Mushroom Jump Starters

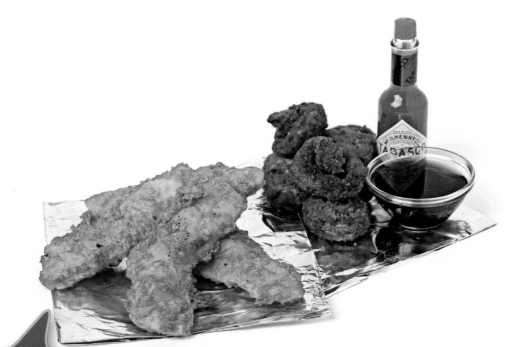

Well, shiver me timbers! Here's some delectable sea-food fare recommended by me, Captain Jorge! Enjoy a lean, tasty fillet with a burst of mushrooms and a Belly Good S/C Value. Dive in!

## BELLY GOOD

S/C Value = 5/2

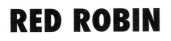

# RED ROBIN

## Apple Harvest Chicken Salad

## BELLY BAD

S/C Value = 27/4

There's a season for everything . . . except this salad. The name may evoke thoughts of autumn and the American ideal, but this plate combines glazed walnuts, apples, and salad dressing for a high sugar value.

# Mighty Caesar with Blackened Chicken Salad

This flavorful salad will sweep you off your feet with juicy chicken and fresh greens drizzled with zesty Caesar dressing. How to order: "Hold the croutons, please."

## BELLY GOOD

S/C Value = 3/2

# RED ROBIN

## Lettuce-Wrapped
## Banzai Burger

## BELLY BAD

S/C Value = 19/4

All lettuce-wrapped burgers are not created equal. The sweet teriyaki marinade and grilled pineapples ramp up the sugar grams to prime your pancreas for one gnarly insulin rush.

# Lettuce-Wrapped Royal Red Robin Burger
## with Mac 'n' Cheese

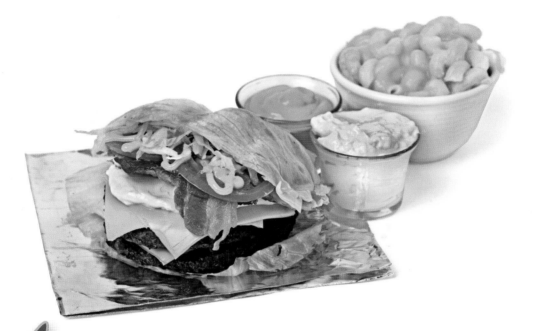

Grab yourself a booth and cozy up to this all-American burger with plenty of flair: crunchy bacon, fresh tomato, and a fried egg wrapped in crisp lettuce. Oh, and did I mention the side of mac and cheese? Enjoy!

## BELLY GOOD

S/C Value = 3/2

## Thai Style Chicken & Rice Noodles

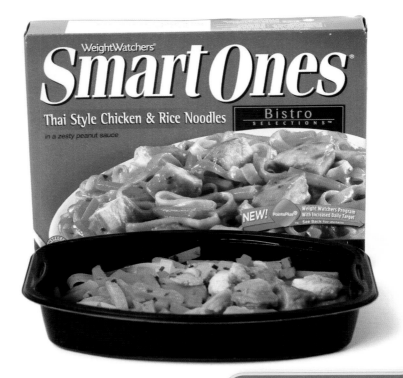

## BELLY BAD

S/C Value = 10/2

> This interpretation of Thai has a sky-high S/C Value, so I'm saying "bye" to this dish. I'll take my chicken in some other form, thank you very much.

# Slow Roasted Turkey Breast

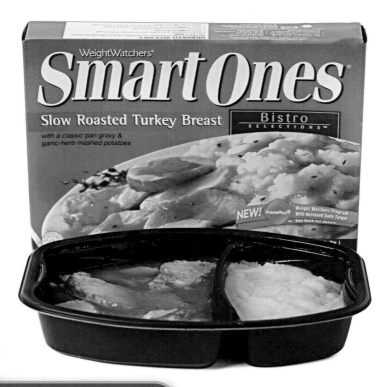

Maybe slow and low wins the race. This tasty, slow-roasted turkey proves to be low in sugar and first in flavor. I'm crowning it the Belly Good champion over its competitor.

## BELLY GOOD

S/C Value = 1/1

## Orange
## Sesame Chicken

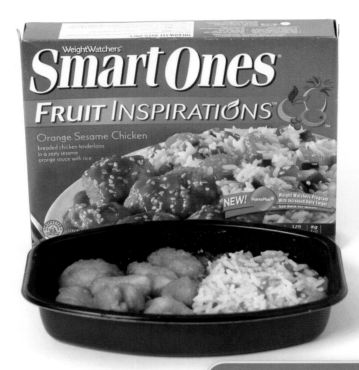

## BELLY BAD

S/C Value = 12/3

You're only as good as the company you keep. In this case, it looks like Chicken has succumbed to the sugary peer pressure of his buddy Orange. Time to find new friends, Chicken . . .

# Broccoli and Cheddar
# Roasted Potatoes

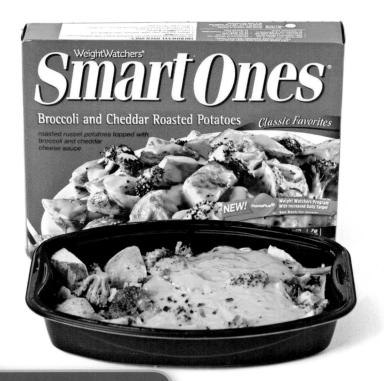

Cheddar is definitely a trigger word for a flavor seeker like me. And right now, all eyes are on this succulent entrée.

## BELLY GOOD

S/C Value = 5/2

# SMART ONES

## Pasta with Ricotta and Spinach

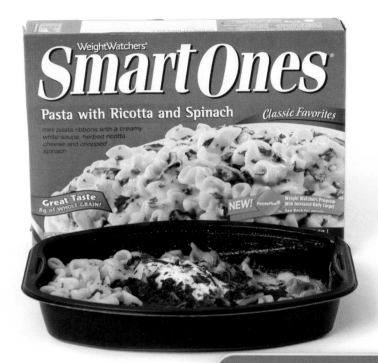

## BELLY BAD

S/C Value = 7/3

If I learned anything as a kid, it's that popping a can of spinach inflates biceps to superhuman size (thanks, Popeye). Unfortunately, the only thing this sugary dish is inflating is your waistline.

# Chicken Parmesan

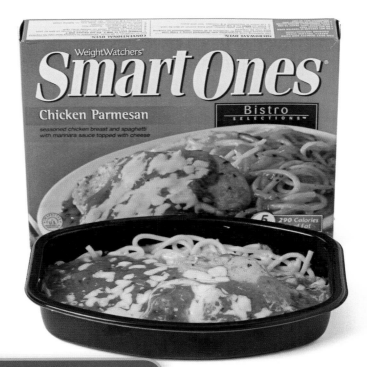

I'm not Italian, but this classic dish has me shouting "Delizioso!" Enjoy lightly breaded Parmesan-crusted chicken and fresh pasta covered in a zesty, low-sugar red sauce.

## BELLY GOOD

S/C Value = 5/2

## Perfect Oatmeal
## with Dried-Fruit Topping

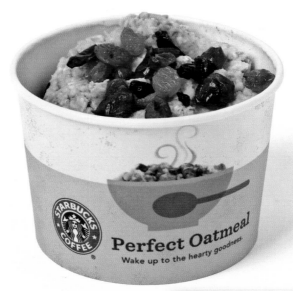

## BELLY BAD

S/C Value = 20/3

One of these things is not like the other . . . and the difference is *fruit*. That tiny handful of dried fruit has 20 grams of sugar ready to heighten your insulin levels. The truth is there's nothing "perfect" about it.

# Perfect Oatmeal with Nut-Medley Topping

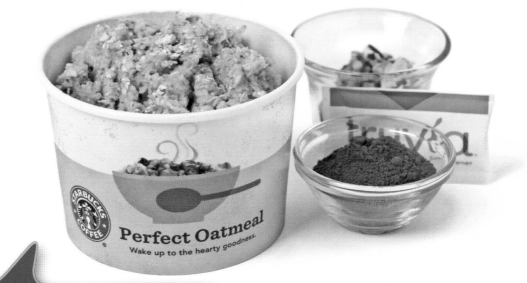

Same illustrious title, only this time it rings true. When your friendly Starbucks barista asks about toppings, simply say: "Mixed nuts" . . . then add some cinnamon and Truvia and go nuts!

## BELLY GOOD

S/C Value = 1/2

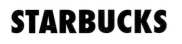

# STARBUCKS

## Reduced-Fat Turkey Bacon, White Cheddar & Cage-Free Egg White Classic Breakfast Sandwich

## BELLY BAD

S/C Value = 6/3

Here again, more "healthy" words that pop off a menu but fall short in the waistline department. Don't start your day on the wrong side of the belly-fat bed.

# Bacon & Gouda Artisan Breakfast Sandwich

**Check out this morning miracle. With only 1 gram of sugar (and a whole lot of taste) you can enjoy crispy bacon, eggs, and melted Gouda, guilt free.**

## BELLY GOOD

S/C Value = 1/2

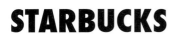

## Protein Artisan
## Snack Plate

## BELLY BAD

S/C Value = 17/2

Only one of these snack plates is getting a rose. The other is going home. After the break . . . okay, I'll just tell you now: it's not this one! I know the outside looks good, but the inside has to match.

# Chicken on Flatbread with Hummus Artisan Snack Plate

Your belly and this snack plate are a match made in heaven. With grilled chicken, crisp cucumbers, hummus, and a lovable S/C Value, I now pronounce you Belly Good . . . you may eat the snack plate!

## BELLY GOOD

S/C Value = 3/2

# STARBUCKS

## Tarragon Chicken Salad Sandwich

## BELLY BAD

S/C Value = 13/3

> Don't let the colorful cranberries and wheat bread fool you into thinking that this is something Mother Nature would approve for your waistline. This sandwich needs a swap.

# Turkey & Swiss Sandwich

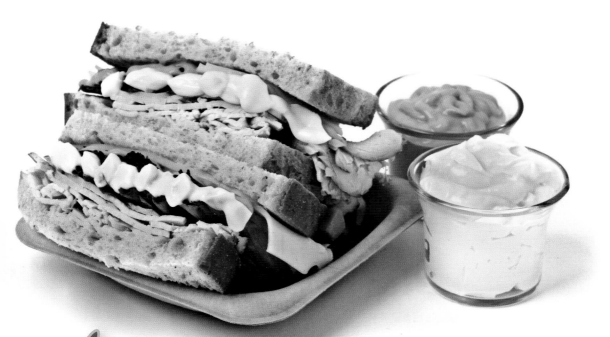

My only complaint is that Starbucks couldn't think of a more exotic name—you know, something European. Nonetheless, this classic combo is a tasty throwback to sunny, summer-day picnics.

## BELLY GOOD

S/C Value = 5/2

# STARBUCKS

## Venti Skinny Iced Latte

## BELLY BAD

S/C Value = 16/1

This frigid mix will ice your belly-fat burn faster than you can say "fat free." I know this can be tough to hear, but milk has sugar. For a slender waistline, we need to reinvent this caffeinated beverage.

# Venti Breve
# Iced Latte

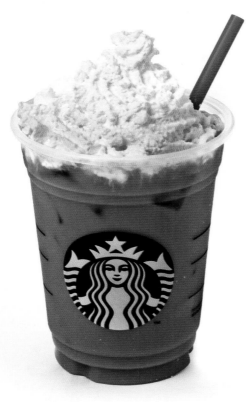

Sip on this sweet, indulgent coffee treat to mesmerize your taste buds and enliven your day. Top with whipped cream. Yum!

## BELLY GOOD

S/C Value = 0/0

# STOUFFER'S

### Chicken à la King

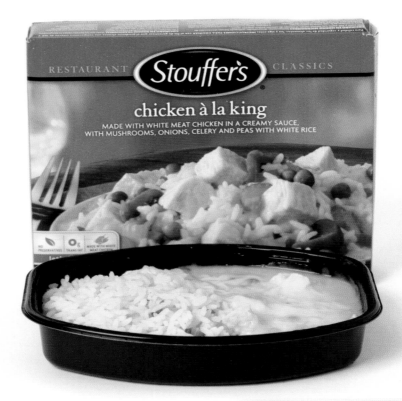

## BELLY BAD

S/C Value = 7/2

King, huh? Maybe king of the plus sizes. This entrée is closer to being a court jester than royalty. Its chicken and veggies might fool your healthy intuition, but the punch line is a high S/C Value.

# Baked Chicken Breast

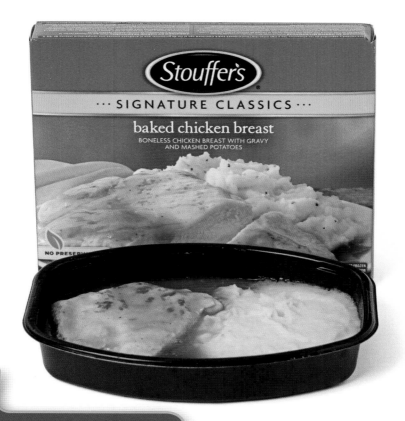

Now here's a ruler of the land with some integrity! With only 1 gram of sugar per serving, let's get this meal a castle and a crown. Jolly good! Or should I say, "Belly Good!"

## BELLY GOOD

S/C Value = 1/1

## Chicken in Barbeque Sauce

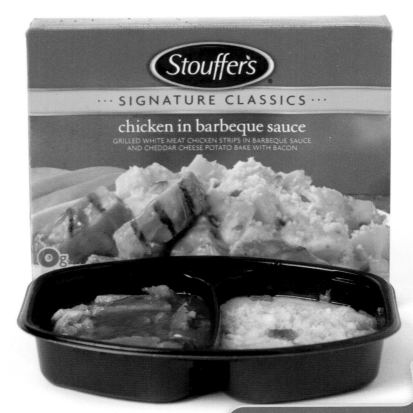

### BELLY BAD

S/C Value = 17/3

Don't bring this to the family barbeque. Believe it or not, this meal has as much sugar as some of the Belly Bad chocolate bars in the back of this book. Nice try, Stouffer's.

# Salisbury Steak

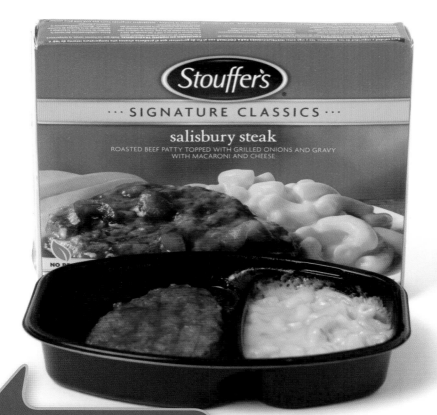

Now we're talkin'!
This mouthwatering steak is enough to make Grandma blush. Add savory mac and cheese to this culinary romance, and you've got yourself a delicious CARB SWAP™.

## BELLY GOOD

S/C Value = 5/2

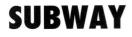

# SUBWAY

## Sunrise Subway Breakfast Melt with Egg Whites

## BELLY BAD

S/C Value = 6/3

Better to let the sun set on this pleasantly titled breakfast choice. Truthfully, the only thing rising will be your waistline measurement if you dive face-first into this sandwich.

# Black Forest Ham,
# Egg & Cheese Muffin Melt

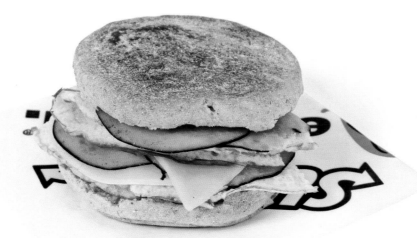

This jump start to your morning will help you cure belly fat with the whole egg, not just the white. You'll easily stay on track with this scrumptious sandwich's exceptional numbers.

## BELLY GOOD

S/C Value = 1/2

# SUBWAY

## Ham on Honey Oat, with Strawberry Yogurt

## BELLY BAD

S/C Value = 19/3

Here's a classic case of "don't judge a book by its cover." There's nothing light or fit about 11 grams of sugar in your yogurt. The honey oat bread is also a major contributor to this meal's high S/C Value.

# Turkey Breast Mini Sub on 9-Grain Wheat with Roasted Chicken Noodle Soup

The reviews are in for this page-turner: "Tasty and trimming!" How to order: "I'll have the Turkey Breast Mini Sub on 9-grain bread and a bowl of chicken noodle soup. On the sandwich I'll have mayo, mustard, lettuce, and tomato."

## BELLY GOOD

S/C Value = 5/2

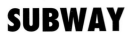
## Sweet Onion
## Chicken Teriyaki 6" Sub

# BELLY BAD

S/C Value = 18/3

> This sweet-by-name sandwich is a cocktail for heightened insulin. Rather than consume a full day's worth of sugar (and then some) plus a handful of carb servings, let's swap it out.

# Chicken Strips on Flatbread

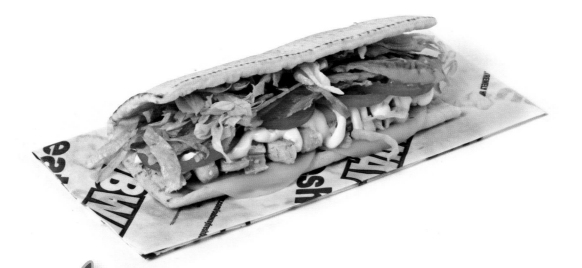

This tasty sandwich is my own creation, so kindly let the sandwich artist know you're building this deliciousness Coach Jorge style! How to order: "I'll have chicken strips on flatbread with provolone, lettuce, tomatoes, and mayonnaise . . . toasted, please!"

**BELLY GOOD**

S/C Value = 2/2

# SUBWAY

## Meatball Marinara
## 6" Sub

## BELLY BAD

S/C Value = 18/4

> Alluring, yes, but this bad boy has something to hide. Sure, its saucy personality may seem fun for a second, but inevitably the romance will be lost in his high-sugar marinara.

# Tuna on Italian White Bread

How to order:
"I'll have the 6" Tuna on Italian, with cheddar cheese and banana peppers." Add freely to taste: mayo, mustard, lettuce, peppers, black olives, salt, and pepper. Toasted? Yes, please!

## BELLY GOOD

S/C Value = 5/2

# TACO BELL

## XXL Grilled Stuft Steak Burrito

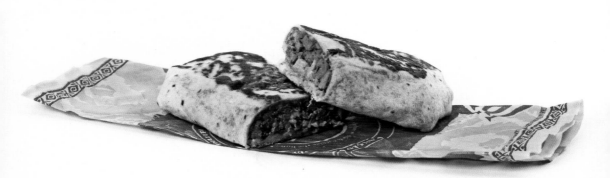

## BELLY BAD

S/C Value = 7/4

I heard the little Chihuahua walked off set when they asked him to promote this grilled, S/C saboteur. Urban legend? Perhaps. But that doesn't change the fact that this burrito is a no-go.

# Chicken Soft Taco
# and Pintos 'n' Cheese

Mmm, I have an epic soft spot for this tasty and trimming duo! How to order: "I'll have the Ranchero Chicken Soft Taco with a side of Pintos 'n' Cheese."

## BELLY GOOD

S/C Value = 3/2

# TACO BELL

## Crunchwrap Supreme

## BELLY BAD

S/C Value = 7/4

This is a definite "no bueno," mis amigos. This crunchy misstep will wrap up your plans for a smaller waistline.

# Crunchy Taco Supreme and Mexican Rice

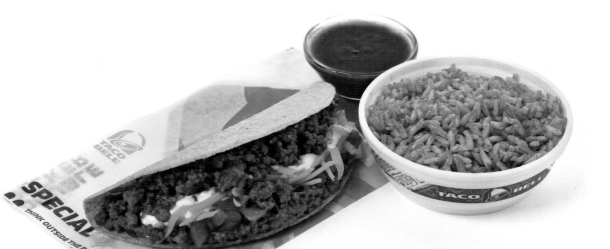

Dear Taco Bell, you are supremely delicious. Your Crunchy Taco is so low in sugar and carbs that I get to add a side of Mexican Rice. I will likely swing by later this week for round two of "awesome." Thanks!

## BELLY GOOD

S/C Value = 2/2

## Volcano Nachos

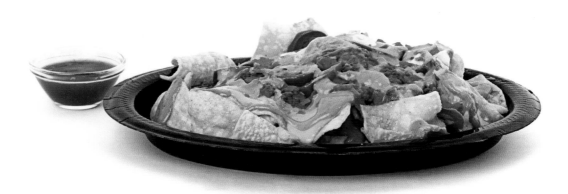

## BELLY BAD

S/C Value = 6/5

> Volcano is right . . .
> your belly will be erupting
> over your waistband
> after munching on this
> natural disaster.

# 3 Fresco Crunchy Tacos with Unsweetened Iced Tea

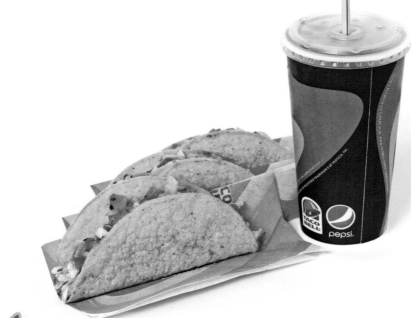

Go ahead and crunch into these tasty tacos, because this meal is worth making some noise about. Talk about serious taste and an exciting S/C Value!

## BELLY GOOD

S/C Value = 3/2

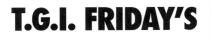

## Sweet & Spicy
## Sesame Chicken

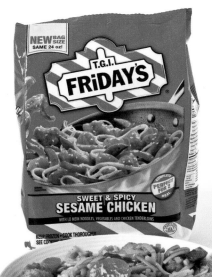

## BELLY BAD

S/C Value = 7/3

There's nothing sweet about this entrée's spicy impact on your belly. This dish is like a Monday— not much to look forward to.

# Creamy Chicken Pasta Carbonara

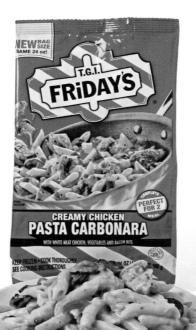

This meal is truly the cream of the crop. There's even bits of bacon in there! Life needs more Fridays . . . and this is a great way to get just that!

## BELLY GOOD

S/C Value = 5/2

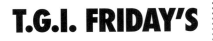

# T.G.I. FRIDAY'S

## Cedar-Seared Salmon Pasta

## BELLY BAD

S/C Value = 34/3

When it comes to this seafood and pasta platter, keep in mind that there's plenty of fish in the sea. With more than two full days' worth of sugar, you definitely want to throw this one back.

# Cajun Shrimp & Chicken Pasta

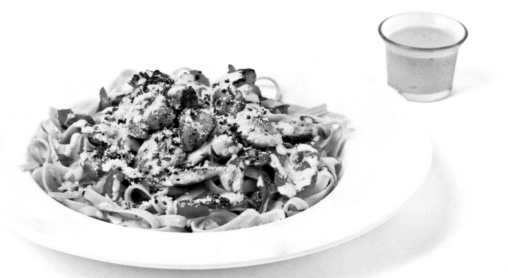

Here's a flavorful Belly Good entrée with enough kick to make you shout "Thank God It's Friday!" What's not to love? Delicious Cajun-style spice is grilled into every blissful bite.

## BELLY GOOD

S/C Value = 4/2

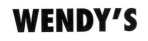
## Apple Pecan Chicken Salad

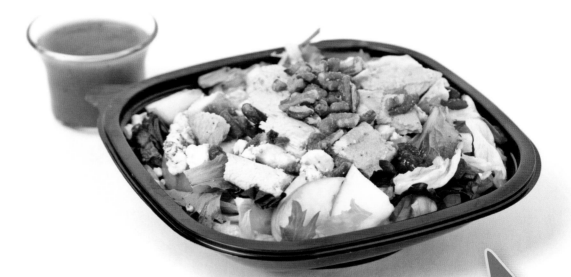

## BELLY BAD

S/C Value = 18/2

By now you've learned that salads can be deceiving. This time Wendy takes a spin on the fruit-o-rama to pump up insulin levels and compromise your weight loss.

# BLT Cobb Salad

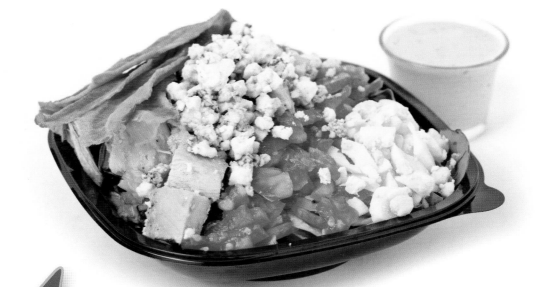

Pile on the flavor without piling on the pounds with this tasty swap. Check out the goods: blue cheese, hardboiled egg, crispy bacon, and avocado-ranch dressing.

## BELLY GOOD

S/C Value = 4/1

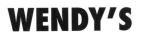

## Ultimate Chicken Grill Sandwich

## BELLY BAD

S/C Value = 9/3

This sandwich is the arch nemesis of its better-loved, Belly Good twin on the next page. Although they appear similar, their qualities are far from identical.

# Crispy Chicken Sandwich

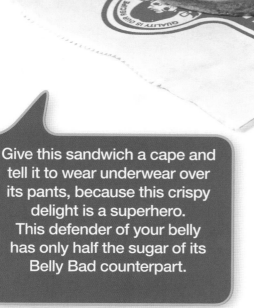

Give this sandwich a cape and tell it to wear underwear over its pants, because this crispy delight is a superhero. This defender of your belly has only half the sugar of its Belly Bad counterpart.

## BELLY GOOD

S/C Value = 4/2

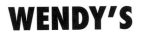

## Baconator Single

## BELLY BAD

S/C Value = 9/3

Don't get me wrong, I love bacon . . . however, this aggressively named Wendy's sandwich will blast your belly-curing plans without batting an eye.

# Jr. Bacon Cheeseburger

Yes, bacon done right! All is forgiven, Wendy, my dear . . . this juicy, bacon sensation is low on sugar and high on taste. Amazing!

## BELLY GOOD

S/C Value = 5/2

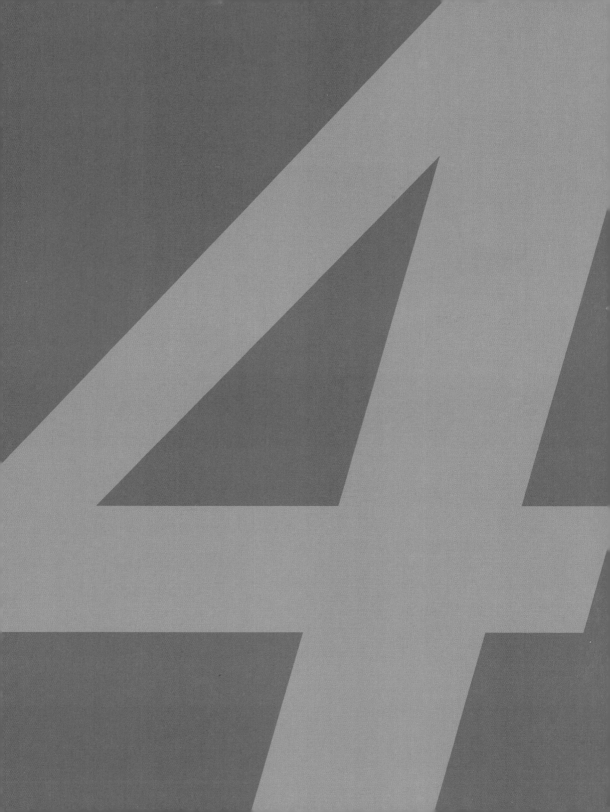

# 4 SWEETENERS

## Alternative Sweeteners

The solution to reducing your sugar intake isn't to use alternative artificial sweeteners such as Sweet'N Low, Equal, or Splenda. You should actually stay away from these because they may cause more harm to your body than good. This chapter will show you how to make your foods sweet without all the sugar. It contains both the Belly Bad sweeteners you should try to avoid and the Belly Good sweeteners I encourage you to start using more often.

The sweeteners that I suggest you avoid are saccharin, aspartame, and sucralose. These are known as *excitotoxins.* This is because they contain neurotransmitters that "overexcite" neurons in the brain, and may cause degeneration and even death in these critical nerve cells.

Saccharin is found in Sweet'N Low. Scientists from the University of Illinois and Boston University have suggested that saccharin be labeled as a carcinogen because they believe that it causes cancer—think about that the next time you reach for one of those tiny pink packets!

Aspartame is in Equal and NutraSweet, as well as thousands of food and drink products like chewing gum and diet soda. Studies have shown that it can cause imbalances in your brain, and it has been proven to negatively affect your nervous system, moods, and quality of sleep. Researchers from Washington University School of Medicine in St. Louis even found a connection between aspartame consumption and seizures.

Sucralose is found in Splenda and is 600 times sweeter than sugar. Sucralose produced significant weight gain in a study at Duke University. Scientists at Duke also found that commonly consumed amounts of sucralose can reduce the amount of "good" gut bacteria by half. Gut bacteria are essential for promoting a healthy digestive system and regular bowel movements. In addition, sucralose contains chlorine—would you want to put something into your body that is used to sanitize pools? Manufactured chlorine compounds like those used in Splenda can cause damage to your organs.

## Smarter Sweetness

You can feel a lot better about the Belly Good sweeteners featured in this chapter. They are approved on the Belly Fat Cure™ because they're all natural. I recommend stevia and xylitol if you want something healthy that tastes truly sweet.

Stevia is an herb that doesn't cause blood-sugar spikes. It's much sweeter than sugar, which means that you don't need a lot to satisfy your sweet tooth. The FDA recently approved refined stevia extract (Rebaudioside A, also known as Reb A or rebiana) for use in food and drink products. You can also purchase whole-leaf stevia; it just has to be labeled as a dietary supplement.

Xylitol, derived from the fiber of fruits and vegetables, is a sugar alcohol. Sugar alcohols add sweetness to foods and drinks without any nutrients. They are neither sugars nor alcohols, despite their name. They're actually carbohydrates, and they don't cause blood-sugar spikes the way regular sugar does because they're converted to glucose more slowly, requiring little or no insulin to be metabolized. This means they cause less disturbance to the endocrine system.

In addition to xylitol, the most popular types of sugar alcohols are maltitol and erythritol. Maltitol is being used in baked goods, chocolates, and cookies more and more. Erythritol is one of the best sugar alcohols you can consume. Found in the stevia-based sweetener Truvia, which you will see in this chapter, it has been found to cause much less intestinal disturbances. The fermentation that can occur when other sugar alcohols are consumed in excess does not occur with erythritol.

On the Belly Fat Cure™, you don't count any grams listed as "sugar alcohols" in the sugar category, but they may be counted on a nutrition label under "total carbohydrates." If this is the case, they're counted as carbs in the S/C Value, but you won't have to track these separately.

In this chapter, most sweeteners have an S/C Value of 0/0. However, some products have an S/C Value of 0/1. Although these are Belly Good, be conscious of how much of these products you use. If you use too much, a product with an S/C Value of 0/0 can then easily have one of 0/1, or a product with an S/C Value of 0/1 can bump up to a 0/2.

You don't have to give up your sweet tooth if you want to lose belly fat. Stick with these sweeteners and losing 4 to 9 lbs. a week will become that much easier!

# LIQUID SWEETENERS

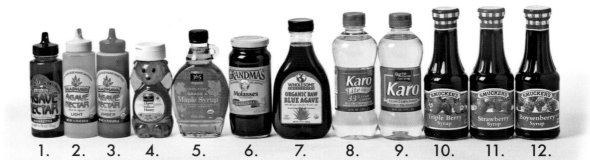

1.    2.    3.    4.    5.    6.    7.    8.    9.    10.    11.    12.

## BELLY BAD

1. Madhava Agave Nectar Amaretto (1 Tbsp.): 15/1
2. Madhava Agave Nectar Light (1 Tbsp.): 16/1
3. Madhava Agave Nectar Amber (1 Tbsp.): 16/1
4. 365 Everyday Value Organic Wildflower Honey (1 Tbsp.): 17/1
5. 365 Everyday Value Organic 100% Pure Grade A Maple Syrup (¼ cup): 53/3
6. Grandma's Original Molasses (1 Tbsp.): 14/1
7. Wholesome Sweeteners Organic Raw Blue Agave (1 Tbsp.): 16/1
8. Karo Lite Syrup (2 Tbsp.): 7/1
9. Karo Light Corn Syrup with Real Vanilla (2 Tbsp.): 10/2
10. Smucker's Triple Berry Syrup (¼ cup): 44/3
11. Smucker's Strawberry Syrup (¼ cup): 44/3
12. Smucker's Boysenberry Syrup (¼ cup): 44/3

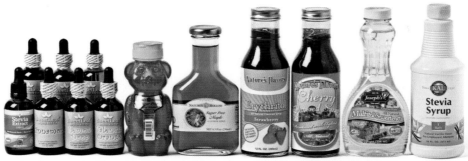

1. through 7.  8.  9.  10.  11.  12.  13.

**BELLY GOOD**

1. 365 Everyday Value Stevia Extract Liquid: 0/0
2. SweetLeaf Liquid Stevia Cinnamon: 0/0
3. SweetLeaf Liquid Stevia Lemon Drop: 0/0
4. SweetLeaf Liquid Stevia Valencia Orange: 0/0
5. SweetLeaf Liquid Stevia Chocolate: 0/0
6. SweetLeaf Liquid Stevia Vanilla Crème: 0/0
7. SweetLeaf Liquid Stevia Peppermint: 0/0
8. Nature's Hollow Sugar Free Honey Substitute (2 Tbsp.): 0/1
9. Nature's Hollow Sugar Free Maple Flavored Syrup (¼ cup): 0/1
10. Nature's Flavors Strawberry Flavored Erythritol Syrup (¼ cup): 0/1
11. Nature's Flavors Cherry Flavored Xylitol Syrup (2 Tbsp.): 0/1
12. Joseph's All Natural Maltitol Sweetener (½ cup): 0/1
13. KAL Stevia Syrup: 0/1

# POWDERED SWEETENERS

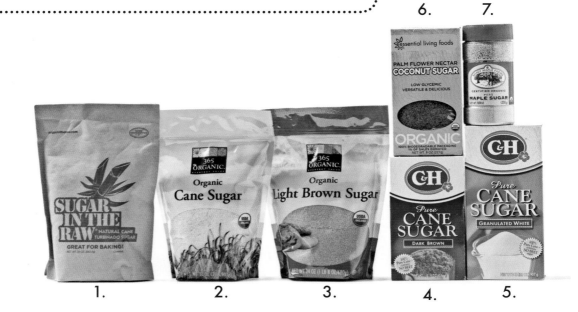

6.    7.

1.    2.    3.    4.    5.

## BELLY BAD

1. Sugar in the Raw Natural Cane Turbinado Sugar (1 tsp.): 4/0
2. 365 Everyday Value Organic Cane Sugar (1 tsp.): 4/0
3. 365 Everyday Value Organic Light Brown Sugar (1 tsp.): 4/0
4. C & H Pure Cane Sugar Dark Brown (1 tsp.): 4/0
5. C & H Pure Cane Sugar Granulated White (1 tsp.): 4/0
6. Essential Living Foods Palm Flower Nectar Coconut Sugar (1 tsp.): 24/2
7. Shady Maple Farms Certified Organic Pure Maple Sugar (1 tsp.): 4/0

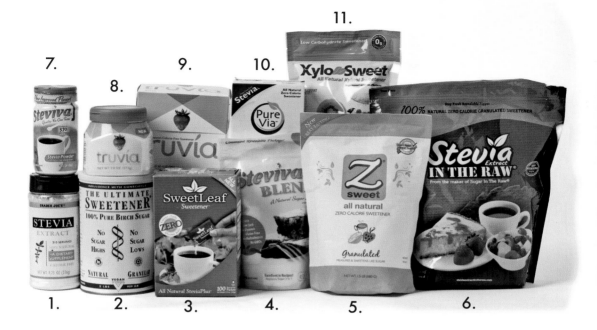

7.    8.    9.    10.    11.

1.    2.    3.    4.    5.    6.

## BELLY GOOD

1. Trader Joe's Stevia Extract: 0/0
2. The Ultimate Sweetener 100% Pure Birch Sugar (xylitol): 0/0
3. SweetLeaf Sweetener: 0/0
4. Steviva Blend: 0/0
5. Z Sweet: 0/0
6. Stevia Extract in the Raw: 0/0
7. Steviva 100% Pure Stevia Powder: 0/0
8. Scoopable Truvia: 0/0
9. Truvia (1 packet): 0/0
10. Pure Via: 0/0
11. Xylo-Sweet (xylitol): 0/0

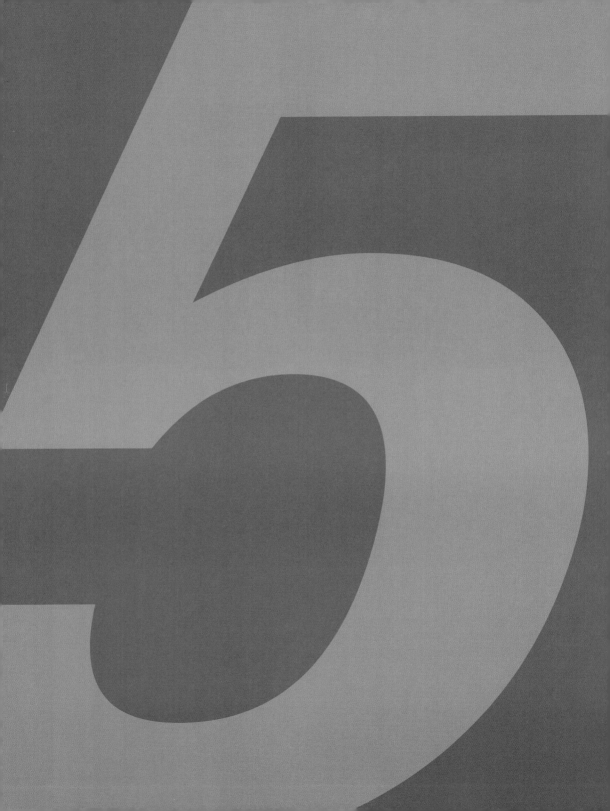

# 5 ICE
# CREAM

## How Sweet It Is

"I can still eat ice cream and lose belly fat?" you ask. The answer is YES! I have a major sweet tooth myself, and I know that if I avoided all sweet treats, I would eventually succumb to temptation and overindulge. In order to keep my cravings in check, I make sure to have a sweet treat every day.

Ice cream is very much a favorite of mine in the "sweet treat" category. However, it's definitely no easy task to track down an all-natural, sugar-free kind. Trust me, as someone who is constantly on the lookout, I consider myself an expert. Fortunately for us both, I've found a couple of delicious brands that are Belly Fat Cure™ approved.

However, before you drive off into the sunset with a pint of ice cream under your arm, please allow me to highlight a couple guidelines. First, I am by no means suggesting that you substitute ice cream for a meal. Yes, that would be delicious. It would also be incredibly unhealthy. Second, these are not freebies. If you want to enjoy ice cream during the day, you must include it when you track your other meals so that you stay within 15/6™.

I hope you enjoy these Belly Good sweet treats just as much as I do!

# ICE CREAM

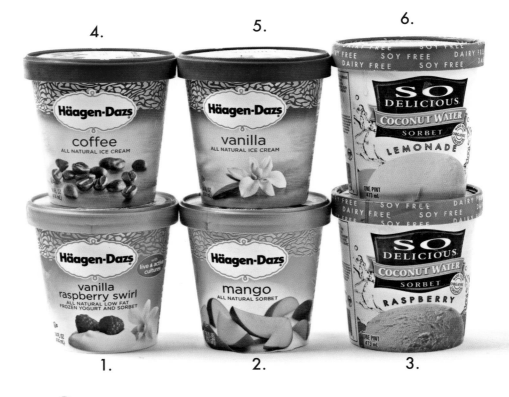

4. 5. 6.

1. 2. 3.

## BELLY BAD

1. Häagen-Dazs Vanilla Raspberry Swirl Frozen Yogurt (½ cup): 54/2
2. Häagen-Dazs Mango Sorbet (½ cup): 36/2
3. So Delicious Coconut Water Raspberry Sorbet (½ cup): 24/2
4. Häagen-Dazs Coffee (½ cup): 21/2
5. Häagen-Dazs Vanilla (½ cup): 21/2
6. So Delicious Coconut Water Lemonade Sorbet (½ cup): 25/2

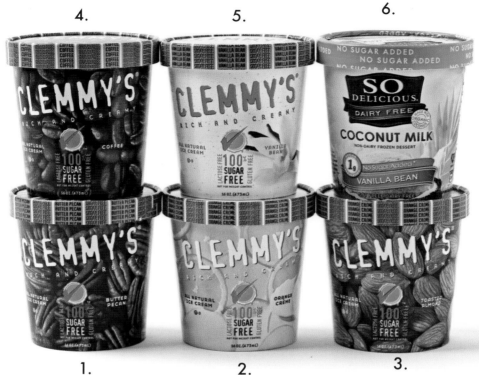

**BELLY GOOD**

1. Clemmy's Butter Pecan (½ cup): 0/1
2. Clemmy's Orange Crème (½ cup): 0/2
3. Clemmy's Toasted Almond (½ cup): 0/2
4. Clemmy's Coffee (½ cup): 0/2
5. Clemmy's Vanilla Bean (½ cup): 0/1
6. So Delicious Dairy Free Coconut Milk No-Sugar Added Vanilla Bean (½ cup): 1/1

# ICE CREAM

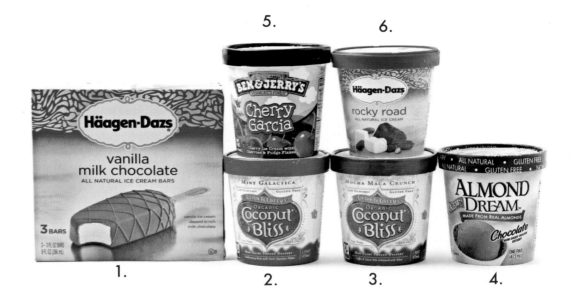

5.

6.

1.

2.

3.

4.

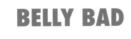

## BELLY BAD

1. Häagen-Dazs Vanilla Milk Chocolate Ice Cream Bars (1): 20/2
2. Luna & Larry's Organic Coconut Bliss Mint Galactica (½ cup): 15/2
3. Luna & Larry's Organic Coconut Bliss Mocha Maca Crunch (½ cup): 13/1
4. Almond Dream Chocolate (½ cup): 18/2
5. Ben & Jerry's Cherry Garcia (½ cup): 23/2
6. Häagen-Dazs Rocky Road (½ cup): 22/2

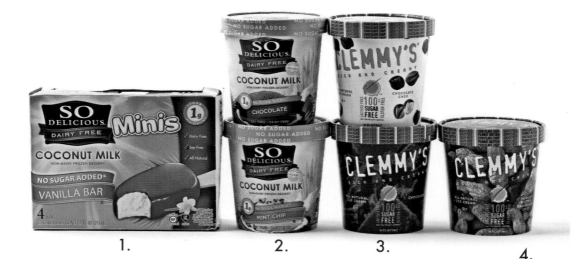

1.

2.

5.

6.

3.

4.

## BELLY GOOD

1. So Delicious Dairy Free Coconut Milk Minis Vanilla Bar (1): 1/1
2. So Delicious Dairy Free Coconut Milk No-Sugar Added Mint Chip (½ cup): 1/1
3. Clemmy's Chocolate (½ cup): 0/2
4. Clemmy's Peanut Butter Chocolate Chip (½ cup): 0/2
5. So Delicious Dairy Free Coconut Milk No-Sugar Added Chocolate (½ cup): 1/1
6. Clemmy's Chocolate Chip (½ cup): 0/2

# ICE CREAM

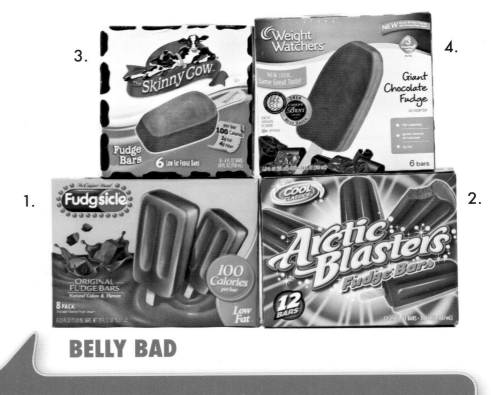

3. The Skinny Cow — Fudge Bars — 6 Low Fat Fudge Bars

4. Weight Watchers — Giant Chocolate Fudge — ice cream bar — 6 bars

1. Fudgsicle — ORIGINAL FUDGE BARS — Natural Colors & Flavors — 8 PACK — 100 Calories per bar — Low Fat

2. COOL CLASSICS — Arctic Blasters — Fudge Bars — 12 BARS

## BELLY BAD

1. Fudgsicle Original Fudge Bars (1): 14/1
2. Cool Classics Arctic Blasters Fudge Bars (1): 14/2
3. Skinny Cow Fudge Bars (1): 13/2
4. Weight Watchers Giant Chocolate Fudge (1): 15/2

## CLEMMY'S ICE CREAM

When it comes to indulgent ice-cream treats that are sweet without the sugar, my absolute favorite is Clemmy's. I recently had the pleasure of meeting the owners of Clemmy's and was blown away by their dedication to creating wholesome, all-natural products. They never use artificial flavors or chemicals to enhance their ice cream. Instead, they churn up delicious flavors and novelties with real cream and tasty, all-natural flavors. That's why I always recommend Clemmy's to clients, friends, and family. My two boys are constantly asking for Clemmy's (they definitely inherited my sweet tooth!) and I love that I can give them ice cream without worrying about their health.

Discover all their magical products at: **ClemmysIceCream.com**.

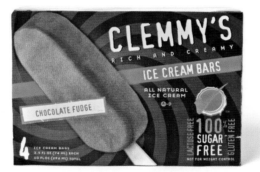

## BELLY GOOD

Clemmy's Chocolate Fudge Ice Cream Bar (1): 0/1

# 6 SODA

I love cracking open a can of soda when I'm on the go. It's such a sweet, refreshing complement to many of the tasty CARB SWAPS™ in this book. I know many of you feel the same way. Still, regular soda is a definite no-go when it comes to curing belly fat. It is by far one of the most common sources of hidden sugar out there. It's a liquid insulin rush in a can!

The dangers of diet soda are less obvious. Many people assume that "diet" means "healthy," and mistakenly drink the stuff every day. In truth, most diet sodas contain harmful artificial sweeteners like sucralose and aspartame (see pages 231 and 232 to learn more about these sweeteners). That's why I swap those sugar-heavy cans and artificial choices with a truly sweet alternative: Zevia.

In my mind, the makers of Zevia are nothing short of miracle workers. How else could they create such sweet, bubbly wonders for me to enjoy every day? And, of course, I absolutely love the fact that they refuse to add hidden sugars or dangerous artificial sweeteners in their products. Part of my mission is to get Zevia into all grocery stores nationwide. Imagine the impact on our nation's health by making this important swap!

Check out all their amazing flavors at: **Zevia.com**. (Cola is my personal favorite!)

# SODA

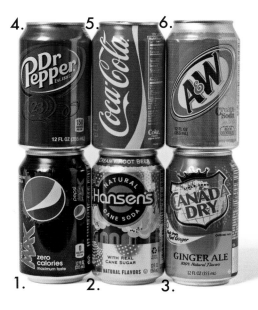

4. 5. 6.

1. 2. 3.

## BELLY BAD

1. Pepsi Max Zero Calories (12 oz.): 0/0*
2. Hansen's Creamy Root Beer (12 oz.): 43/3
3. Canada Dry Ginger Ale (12 oz.): 25/2
4. Dr Pepper (12 oz.): 40/2
5. Coca-Cola (12 oz.): 39/2
6. A & W Cream Soda (12 oz.): 44/3

*but contains aspartame*

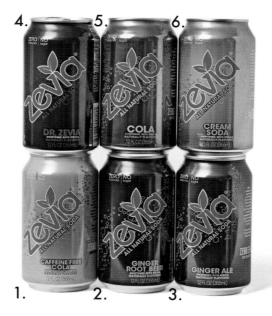

## BELLY GOOD

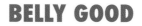

1. Zevia Caffeine Free Cola (12 oz.): 0/1
2. Zevia Ginger Root Beer (12 oz.): 0/1
3. Zevia Ginger Ale (12 oz.): 0/1
4. Zevia Dr. Zevia (12 oz.): 0/1
5. Zevia Cola (12 oz.): 0/1
6. Zevia Cream Soda (12 oz.): 0/1

# SODA

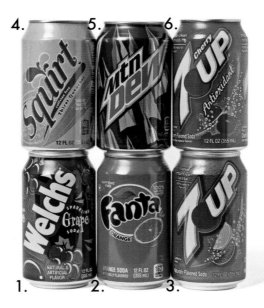

4. 5. 6.

1. 2. 3.

## BELLY BAD

1. Welch's Sparkling Grape Soda (12 oz.): 51/3
2. Fanta Orange (12 oz.): 44/3
3. 7UP (12 oz.): 38/2
4. Squirt (12 oz.): 38/2
5. Mountain Dew (12 oz.): 46/3
6. Cherry 7UP Antioxidant (12 oz.): 38/2

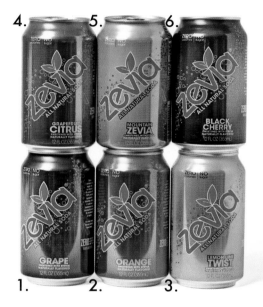

## BELLY GOOD

1. Zevia Grape (12 oz.): 0/1
2. Zevia Orange (12 oz.): 0/1
3. Zevia Lemon Lime Twist (12 oz.): 0/1
4. Zevia Grapefruit Citrus (12 oz.): 0/1
5. Zevia Mountain Zevia (12 oz.): 0/1
6. Zevia Black Cherry (12 oz.): 0/1

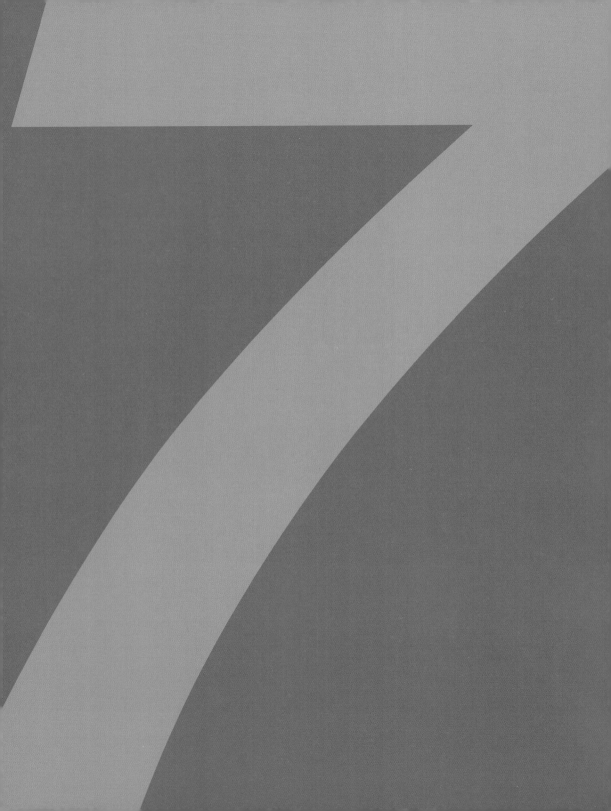

# 7

## Bonus Chapter
# MEAL-REPLACEMENT BARS

Some days I find myself so busy that I don't even have time to cruise through a drive-thru for a tasty CARB SWAP™. I know it's best to eat three fresh, balanced meals every day; however, I also know the reality of my life. I'm often in a hurry! I cannot stress enough the importance of always being prepared. If I'm not equipped with a meal-replacement bar when I rush out the door each morning, I might skip a meal and be tempted to veer off track later in the day. That's why I've learned to carry with me one of my favorite, thinkThin meal-replacement bars, at all times.

I should be more specific. When I say "favorite," I actually mean "only."

The thinkThin protein bars are the only meal-replacement bars I eat. Why? Well, first of all—this should come as no surprise—they're 100 percent delicious! They have a tasty selection of indulgent flavors such as creamy peanut butter, chocolate-covered strawberries, and lemon pie. Second, thinkThin bars are completely sugar free. They sweeten their bars with maltitol, which is a safe, Belly Fat Cure™–approved sugar alcohol.

If you're a super-busy person like me, I recommend you pick your favorites and make sure to have one on hand next time you're in a hurry.

# MEAL-REPLACEMENT BARS

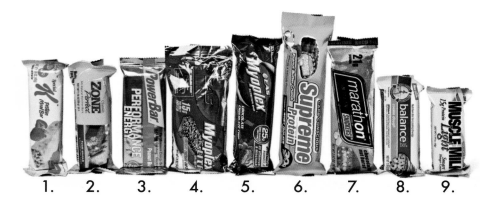

1.  2.  3.  4.  5.  6.  7.  8.  9.

## BELLY BAD

1. Special K Strawberry Protein Meal Bar: 15/2
2. Zone Perfect Fudge Graham Bar: 15/2
3. PowerBar Performance Energy Peanut Butter: 26/3
4. EAS Myoplex Lite Chocolate Chocolate Chip Crisp Bar: 11/2
5. EAS Myoplex Chocolate Chocolate Chip Nutrition Bar: 14/2
6. Supreme Protein Peanut Butter Crunch: 10/2
7. Snickers Marathon Protein Bar Chocolatey Nut Burst: 18/2
8. Balance Bar Cookie Dough: 17/2
9. Muscle Milk Light Bar Chocolate Peanut Caramel: 9/1

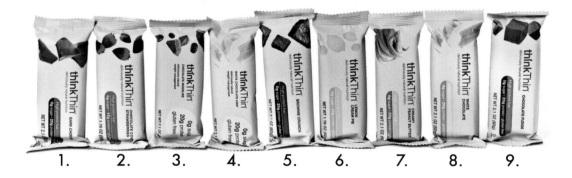

## BELLY GOOD

1. thinkThin Dark Chocolate: 0/2
2. thinkThin Chocolate Covered Strawberries: 0/2
3. thinkThin Chocolate Mudslide: 0/2
4. thinkThin White Chocolate Chip: 0/2
5. thinkThin Brownie Crunch: 0/2
6. thinkThin Lemon Cream Pie: 0/2
7. thinkThin Creamy Peanut Butter: 0/2
8. thinkThin White Chocolate: 0/2
9. thinkThin Chocolate Fudge: 0/2

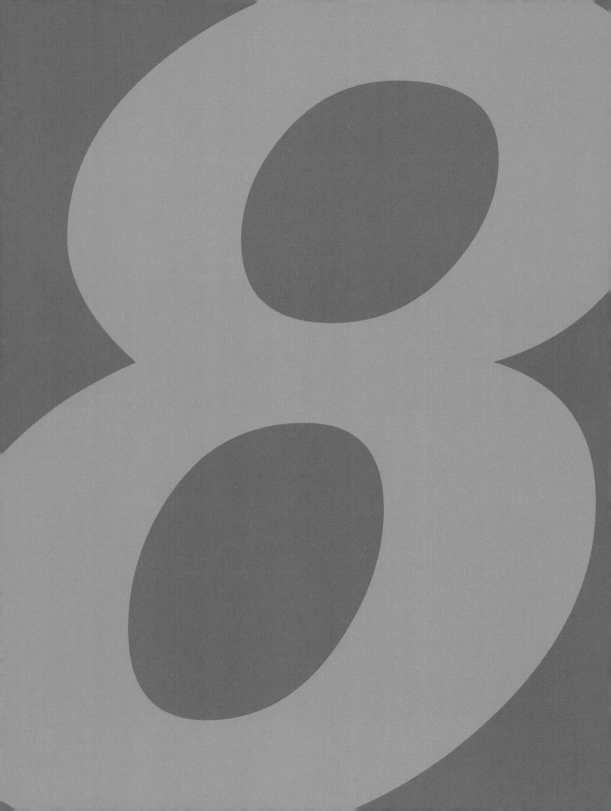

# 8 Frequently Asked Questions (FAQs)

**1. How do the meals in this book differ from those suggested in the original *Belly Fat Cure*™ book?**

In the original *Belly Fat Cure*™, most of the Belly Good meals are healthy, make-it-yourself "do overs" to replace a familiar meal from a fast-food chain, restaurant, or frozen entrée. By comparison, the majority of Belly Good meals in this book are a healthier choice from the same chain or restaurant as the Belly Bad choice. Now that little to no preparation is required on your part, the meals are even more convenient (and still delicious!).

**2. Is it healthy to frequently eat on the go?**

Yes, if you make smart decisions. Fast food has become detrimental to many Americans' health because they do not make the right choices. Most meals at fast-food chains and restaurants (as well as frozen meals) are loaded with hidden sugar and carbs. However, the Belly Good choices in this book are perfectly acceptable. We've done the difficult work for you, so there's no need to guess about healthy options the next time you're out.

### 3. Is it bad to eat Quick Meals every day?

While I still suggest eating fresh foods as much as possible, every Quick Meal featured in this book is designed to keep your S/C Value on track, and therefore fine to eat frequently.

### 4. When should I begin to see weight-loss results?

If you follow the plan exactly and keep your daily intake at an S/C Value of 15/6™ or less, you should see weight-loss results after just one week. Many of my clients begin to see a smaller waist within a matter of days!

### 5. Why are some S/C Values different from the restaurant's description?

All nutritional information in this book was accurate as this book went to press. However, restaurants may have updated their information since then. If you suspect that an S/C Value is outdated, I encourage you to visit the restaurant's website directly to cross-reference. If our numbers need to be updated, please visit **JorgeCruise .com** and let us know!

### 6. Where can I find the S/C Value of other meals from popular restaurants and fast-food chains?

*The Belly Fat Cure*™ *Sugar & Carb Counter* contains the S/C Value for hundreds of meals in the "dining out" section. But even if you don't find the specific meal you're looking for, this book shows you how to easily calculate the S/C Value of a meal yourself.

### 7. What general guidelines do you have for ordering other meals when I'm on the go?

— I recommend that you keep to the CARB SWAPS™ in this book when eating on the go so that you're sure to be sticking to the correct S/C Value. But there are some general guidelines that you can follow if you're at a restaurant without the options from this book. You definitely don't want to find yourself lost with no idea what to order.

— Pay close attention to descriptions on menus. You've learned from this book that some meals from fast-food chains and restaurants appear to be healthy but are not due to the way they're prepared. For example, many seemingly safe salads are actually poor choices because the dressings put on them are loaded with hidden sugars and dangerous artificial sweeteners like sucralose. Don't be afraid to order a salad with a dressing other than the one listed on the menu, or ask for it on the side so that you can control the amount. Burgers can also be a great option, if you order them without the bun.

— Become more aware of certain terms on menus. For example, "grilled" chicken is always a healthier choice than "fried." Also, don't let "fat free" fool you. A fat-free muffin, for instance, may contain a ton of sugar. Finally, one of the key ways to stay at or below your daily S/C Value of 15/6™ is to drink water, green tea, or unsweetened iced tea with your meal instead of sugary soda.

## 8. Can I be a vegetarian on this plan?

Of course you can! You'll follow the Belly Fat Cure™ by simply substituting meats with your own preferred vegetarian (or vegan) options. If you decide to

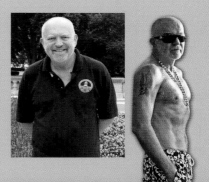

## Ken lost 60 lbs.

Age: 62
Height: 6'3"
Belly Inches Lost: 7

Jorge's programs have inspired me to permanently change my lifestyle. I started with his 8 Minutes in the Morning program and soon discovered the Belly Fat Cure™. I combined 15/6™ tracking with daily walking and dropped 60 lbs and 7 inches off my waist in the first year. Gradually, my blood pressure, cholesterol, and blood glucose lowered from medically dangerous to normal levels.

I haven't brought Belly Bad foods into my home in two years. I look and feel younger and have lots of energy. I'm a happy, healthy 62-year-old and proud of it!

### BEST TIP FOR SUCCESS:

First, remove all Belly Bad foods from your pantry and refrigerator and restock with Belly Good products. Then track, track, track! Wise food choices will become a way of life reinforced by the way you look and feel.

use meat substitutes, be sure to correctly calculate the sugar and carb content of all foods. One word of caution: carbohydrates often become the dominant source of energy in a vegetarian lifestyle. Be sure that the majority of your carbs come from vegetables, and you're taking in the appropriate fats from non-animal sources (such as avocados, olive oil, and nuts).

### 9. Will this plan work for my whole family?

Yes, the Belly Fat Cure™ is a healthy lifestyle for absolutely everyone. Monitoring hidden sugar is important for the overall health of children, teens, adults, and seniors, regardless of gender or body weight.

### 10. Is this program safe for my kids?

Definitely! Limiting sugar in your children's diet and replacing it with smarter options will increase overall health, both inside and out. Low-sugar, nutrient-rich foods are as equally beneficial for your kids as they are for you.

It may be difficult to change your kids' minds about sugar if they've fallen into a habit of constantly eating sugary snacks. Please do not let this discourage you from guiding them to a healthier lifestyle. I suggest that you lead by example first. Then get your children involved by teaching them about the benefits of certain foods and letting them help you prepare snacks and meals. Your kids will be more interested in the foods they're eating if they help create the meals with you. Try to make cooking something fun you and your kids can enjoy together.

### 11. What kinds of artificial sweeteners should I avoid?

As I mentioned earlier in the book, the main artificial sweeteners that you should try to avoid are aspartame (which is found in Equal and NutraSweet), sucralose (found in Splenda), and saccharin (found in Sweet'N Low). These substances are unhealthy because they are excitotoxins. This means that they "overexcite" neurons in the brain, causing degeneration and even death in important nerve cells. When too many nerve cells die, your nervous system begins to malfunction, and it is unable to communicate with other parts of your body. This can ultimately lead to

Parkinson's disease, multiple sclerosis, and Alzheimer's disease, among other nervous-system disorders. Sucralose is also dangerous because of its chlorine properties.

## 12. Do sugar alcohols count toward the S/C Value?

Sugar alcohols don't actually contain any sugar or alcohol. They're a type of carbohydrate that requires very little insulin to be converted into energy. Sugar alcohols are used in foods for sweetness but don't cause a major spike in blood sugar or affect your immune system in any way. Any grams listed as "sugar alcohols" do not count as sugar on the S/C Value. Sugar alcohols may, however, be included on a label under "total carbohydrates," which means that they'll be counted as carbs on the S/C Value. There is no need to keep track of these separately.

Please note: Some people find that they get an upset stomach after consuming sugar alcohols. Tolerance varies from person to person. Excessive amounts of sugar alcohols may lead to unwanted bloating, yet in moderation, they shouldn't cause digestive issues. Pay attention to your own personal level of tolerance.

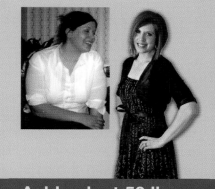

## Ashlee lost 50 lbs.

Age: 31

Height: 5'7"

Belly Inches Lost: 8

During the first few years of marriage, I gained 50 pounds. On top of that, I struggled with infertility. I thought to myself, *What kind of a woman am I if I can't carry a child?* I felt sad and worthless and began eating to try to curb the pain. There were several moments when I found myself eating and sobbing at the same time. I would eat until I was sick, and then feel guilty for eating so much.

Around this time, I picked up *8 Minutes in the Morning for Real Shapes, Real Sizes,* and decided to give it a whirl. Shortly after, I read *The Belly Fat Cure™.* I couldn't believe how much sugar I was eating! I still enjoy my treats, but only in moderation. I'm back to the weight I was on my wedding day, and I'm free to be happy again. Thank you, Jorge, for helping restore my confidence and hope in life!

### BEST TIP FOR SUCCESS:

Keep a journal of your weight-loss journey. Losing weight affects you emotionally as much as physically. Write down your goals, vent your frustrations, and celebrate your victories!

### 13. Why isn't fiber taken into account?

I assure you, the fiber is there. However, this program is all about keeping things simple. Including both vegetables and whole grains in your meals will allow you to consume a healthy amount of fiber. To fully understand your digestive system, please refer to Chapter 3 of *The Belly Fat Cure™ Fast Track*.

### 14. Is it bad to eat the same meals over and over?

Absolutely not! If you prefer certain meals to others that keep your S/C Value on track, and you enjoy eating them often, go right ahead. Many of my most successful clients automate their meals. However, I do find it beneficial to occasionally vary your meals so that you don't grow bored and stray off track.

### 15. Can I still drink alcohol on this program?

Yes, you can enjoy adult beverages in moderation (I suggest a glass of wine in the evening). However, if you find that you're not losing weight on this program, I recommend avoiding alcohol completely.

### 16. Should I still keep track of how many calories I'm eating?

This program is different from other weight-loss plans because it does not focus on counting calories. I strongly believe that counting calories is not the most effective way to moderate your eating and lose belly fat. Simply apply the S/C Value to your daily diet and you will be successful in your weight loss.

### 17. Can I use the original *Belly Fat Cure™* in addition to this book?

Absolutely! In fact, I encourage you to use both books as resources to learn which meals work best for you. The "do overs" I suggest in *The Belly Fat Cure™* can be substituted for the on-the-go CARB SWAPS™ in this book. Again, I find it best to vary your diet so that you're always tantalizing your taste buds every waking day.

### 18. Does *Quick Meals* work hand in hand with *The Belly Fat Cure™ Fast Track?*

The Fast Track is a 14-day program that follows a specific menu to accelerate weight loss by using the Ultimate Carb Swap™. In contrast, this book focuses on the core principal of the Belly Fat Cure™: 15/6™. If you would like to accelerate your belly fat loss in just 2 weeks, I recommend consulting *The Belly Fat Cure™ Fast Track*.

### 19. Should I be worried about my cholesterol levels increasing on this program?

If you have high cholesterol, I recommend speaking with your doctor before starting any weight-loss plan. However, it's more likely that the Belly Fat Cure™ will help lower your cholesterol rather than raise it. In fact, some studies reveal sugar as the largest contributor to high cholesterol. Many sugars travel directly to your liver and get converted to fat, which is sent into your blood, increasing your LDL levels (otherwise known as bad cholesterol). For more information and research, please see *The Belly Fat Cure™* and *The Belly Fat Cure™ Fast Track*.

### 20. Should I be worried about the amount of sodium found in frozen meals?

If you have high blood pressure, one of the best things you can do for your body is to reduce your belly fat. That being said, frozen meals may not be your best option, as many contain higher sodium levels than fresh foods do. Consult the nutrition labels on frozen meals to see which ones contain the least amount of sodium, but also consider some of the non-frozen Belly Good meals.

### 21. Do frozen meals contain any chemicals and preservatives that I should be concerned about?

Some studies have shown that frozen meals can contain chemicals and preservatives that inhibit maximum health. However, the frozen meals I suggest in this book contain less of these additives. If you're concerned, remember that there's no need to consume any frozen meals. Simply select another Belly Good meal from this book.

### 22. What brands of frozen meals do you suggest?

*The Belly Fat Cure™ Sugar & Carb Counter* contains the S/C Value of hundreds of frozen meals. However, not all are Belly Good. Please review the list carefully to select a healthy option.

### 23. How much should I exercise on this program in order to lose weight?

Despite what you're constantly told, research shows that exercise can actually be counterproductive to weight loss. If you run on the treadmill for hours, you may burn a lot of calories, but it's likely that you will be much hungrier afterward. This makes it difficult to consume the right amount of food necessary for weight loss.

Many of my clients do not exercise at all to lose weight, though they often find that exercise helps them feel even better about themselves. Or they incorporate exercise after they have their diet mastered. If you do want to incorporate exercise into this program, I recommend power walking for 20 minutes each day. It's best to do this in the morning before you've eaten anything. To learn more about the right intensity, see Chapter 7 of *The Belly Fat Cure*™. You can find tips for toning your abs in this chapter as well. And you can also find helpful information about fitness in Chapter 8 of *The Belly Fat Cure*™ *Fast Track.*

### 24. How can I share with you about the weight I've lost?

I'm always eager to hear about the success my clients have on this program. I encourage you to share your story together with before-and-after photos on my Facebook page: **Facebook.com/JorgeCruise.**

### 25. How can I stay updated on upcoming books and other news?

Visit my website (**JorgeCruise.com**) for useful menus and advice. This is the best place to discover new information about upcoming books.

### 26. What if I don't begin to lose weight right away on this program?

There may be something that is stimulating insulin in your food. Be sure to check all dressings, sauces, and drinks you are consuming for sugar or artificial sweeteners. You can also refer to *The Belly Fat Cure*™ *Fast Track* book to help you break through any plateaus.

## 27. Why do I turn to food whenever I'm feeling depressed, frustrated, or anxious?

You're not the only one! Many of my clients confess their biggest hindrance to losing belly fat is emotional eating. I'm sure you've been there: after a bad day, you reach for a sugary snack for comfort to numb the pain. Many of you have acquired an addiction to sugar over the years, making it the first thing you reach for when life is difficult to handle. And it's not an easy thing to overcome. Consult Chapter 7 of *The Belly Fat Cure*™ *Fast Track* or my book *Stubborn Fat Gone!* to learn more about reasons for this addiction and strategies to overcome it.

## 28. How can I make a difference?

The most effective way to influence others in a profound way is to simply spread the message of the Belly Fat Cure™ to family, friends, and co-workers. The transformative impact on your own life will inspire others to choose a healthier lifestyle themselves.

# Index of Meals

**BEEF & PORK**

Applebee's Asiago Peppercorn Steak . . . . . . . . . .27

Boston Market Brisket, Garlicky Lemon
Spinach, and Loaded Mashed Potatoes. . . . .39

Chili's Classic Sirloin, and Spicy Garlic
& Lime Grilled Shrimp . . . . . . . . . . . . . . . . . . . .61

Chipotle Tacos with Corn Tortillas. . . . . . . . . . . . .71

Healthy Choice Café Steamers Roasted
Beef Merlot. . . . . . . . . . . . . . . . . . . . . . . . . . . .91

Lean Cuisine Salisbury Steak with Macaroni
and Cheese. . . . . . . . . . . . . . . . . . . . . . . . . . .121

Olive Garden Parmesan-Crusted Bistecca . . . . . .157

Panda Express Broccoli Beef, Mixed Veggies,
and Fried Rice. . . . . . . . . . . . . . . . . . . . . . . . .159

Stouffer's Salisbury Steak . . . . . . . . . . . . . . . . . . .205

Taco Bell 3 Fresco Crunchy Tacos
with Unsweetened Iced Tea . . . . . . . . . . . . . .219

Taco Bell Crunchy Taco Supreme and
Mexican Rice . . . . . . . . . . . . . . . . . . . . . . . . . .217

**BEVERAGES**

Venti Breve Iced Latte. . . . . . . . . . . . . . . . . . . . . . .201

**BREAKFAST**

Burger King Breakfast Burrito with Sausage,
Egg, Cheese & Salsa, and Regular Iced
Coffee with Cream. . . . . . . . . . . . . . . . . . . . . . .43

Burger King Sausage, Egg & Cheese
Croissan'wich, and Coffee with Cream. . . . . .41

Chick-fil-A Sausage Breakfast Burrito . . . . . . . . . .55

Denny's Ultimate Omelette with Side of
Hash Browns . . . . . . . . . . . . . . . . . . . . . . . . . . .73

Einstein Bros Bagels Nova Lox on an
Everything Bagel Thin, with Americano. . . . . .87

IHOP Bacon Temptation Omelette . . . . . . . . . . . . .97

Jack in the Box Supreme Croissant, and
Coffee with Cream. . . . . . . . . . . . . . . . . . . . . .101

McDonald's Bacon, Egg & Cheese Biscuit . . . . . .143

McDonald's Egg McMuffin . . . . . . . . . . . . . . . . . .141

Panera Breakfast Power Sandwich and
Coffee with Cream. . . . . . . . . . . . . . . . . . . . . .169

Starbucks Bacon & Gouda Artisan Breakfast
Sandwich . . . . . . . . . . . . . . . . . . . . . . . . . . . . .195

Starbucks Perfect Oatmeal with Nut-Medley
Topping . . . . . . . . . . . . . . . . . . . . . . . . . . . . . .193

**BURGERS AND SANDWICHES**

Arby's Jr. Chicken Sandwich with Chopped
Side Salad. . . . . . . . . . . . . . . . . . . . . . . . . . . . .31

Arby's Medium Roast Beef Sandwich . . . . . . . . . .33

Carl's Jr. Low-Carb Portobello Burger . . . . . . . . . .47

Denny's Club Sandwich . . . . . . . . . . . . . . . . . . . . .75

Einstein Bros Bagels Turkey-Breast Deli
Sandwich on Challah. . . . . . . . . . . . . . . . . . . . .89

Jack in the Box Sourdough Grilled-
Chicken Club . . . . . . . . . . . . . . . . . . . . . . . . . .105

Jack in the Box Sourdough Steak Melt . . . . . . . . .103

KFC Ultimate Cheese KFC Snacker . . . . . . . . . . . 113

McDonald's Filet-O-Fish . . . . . . . . . . . . . . . . . . . .149

McDonald's McChicken Sandwich. . . . . . . . . . . . .147

Panera Half Asiago Roast Beef Sandwich
and Half a Classic Salad . . . . . . . . . . . . . . . . .165

Quiznos Alpine Chicken Flatbread Sammie
with Small Broccoli Cheese Soup . . . . . . . . .177

Red Robin Lettuce-Wrapped Royal Red
Robin Burger with Mac 'n' Cheese. . . . . . . . .185

Starbucks Turkey & Swiss Sandwich . . . . . . . . . .199

Subway Chicken Strips on Flatbread . . . . . . . . . .211

Subway Tuna on Italian White Bread. . . . . . . . . . .213

Subway Turkey Breast Mini Sub on 9-Grain Wheat
with Roasted Chicken Noodle Soup . . . . . . .209

Wendy's Crispy Chicken Sandwich . . . . . . . . . . .227

Wendy's Jr. Bacon Cheeseburger. . . . . . . . . . . . . .229

## BURRITOS, FAJITAS & TACOS

Chevy's Lunch Value Original Famous
　　Chicken Fajitas. . . . . . . . . . . . . . . . . . . . . . . . .53

Chili's Chicken Fajitas. . . . . . . . . . . . . . . . . . . . . .65

Chipotle Tacos with Corn Tortillas. . . . . . . . . . . . . .71

Taco Bell 3 Fresco Crunchy Tacos with
　　Unsweetened Iced Tea . . . . . . . . . . . . . . . . . .219

Taco Bell Chicken Soft Taco and Pintos
　　'n' Cheese. . . . . . . . . . . . . . . . . . . . . . . . . . .215

Taco Bell Crunchy Taco Supreme and
　　Mexican Rice . . . . . . . . . . . . . . . . . . . . . . . . .217

## FISH & SEAFOOD

Applebee's Dynamite Shrimp . . . . . . . . . . . . . . . . .23

Applebee's Grilled Shrimp 'N Spinach Salad . . . . .25

Chili's Classic Sirloin, and Spicy Garlic & Lime
　　Grilled Shrimp. . . . . . . . . . . . . . . . . . . . . . . . .61

Chili's Grilled Salmon with Garlic & Herbs . . . . . . .63

Lean Cuisine Lemon Garlic Shrimp. . . . . . . . . . . .125

Lean Cuisine Lemon Pepper Fish . . . . . . . . . . . . .119

Lean Cuisine Salmon with Basil. . . . . . . . . . . . . . .123

Long John Silver's 6-Piece Battered Shrimp
　　with 2 Hush Puppies . . . . . . . . . . . . . . . . . . . .129

Long John Silver's Freshside Grille Salmon
　　Entrée with Lobster Bites . . . . . . . . . . . . . . . .131

McDonald's Filet-O-Fish . . . . . . . . . . . . . . . . . . . .149

Panda Express Crispy Shrimp with Mixed
　　Veggies . . . . . . . . . . . . . . . . . . . . . . . . . . . . . .161

Red Robin Arctic Cod with Mushroom
　　Jump Starters. . . . . . . . . . . . . . . . . . . . . . . . .181

T.G.I. Friday's Cajun Shrimp & Chicken Pasta . . . .223

## MEATLESS

Amy's Brown Rice, Black-Eyed Peas
　　& Veggies Bowl. . . . . . . . . . . . . . . . . . . . . . . . .21

Amy's Indian Palak Paneer. . . . . . . . . . . . . . . . . . .19

Amy's Vegetable Lasagna . . . . . . . . . . . . . . . . . . .17

Chipotle Vegetarian Burrito Bowl . . . . . . . . . . . . . .67

DiGiornio Cheese-Stuffed Crust,
　　Four-Cheese Pizza. . . . . . . . . . . . . . . . . . . . . .77

Kashi Pesto Pasta Primavera. . . . . . . . . . . . . . . . .111

Olive Garden Stuffed Mushrooms
　　and Red Wine. . . . . . . . . . . . . . . . . . . . . . . . .151

Smart Ones Broccoli and Cheddar
　　Roasted Potatoes . . . . . . . . . . . . . . . . . . . . . .189

## PASTA

Amy's Vegetable Lasagna . . . . . . . . . . . . . . . . . . .17

Kashi Chicken Pasta Pomodoro . . . . . . . . . . . . . .109

Kashi Pesto Pasta Primavera. . . . . . . . . . . . . . . . .111

Lean Cuisine Lemon Garlic Shrimp. . . . . . . . . . . .125

Smart Ones Chicken Parmesan . . . . . . . . . . . . . .191

TGI Friday's Creamy Chicken Pasta Carbonara . . .221

TGI Friday's Cajun Shrimp & Chicken Pasta . . . . .223

## PIZZA

DiGiornio Cheese-Stuffed Crust,
　　Four-Cheese Pizza. . . . . . . . . . . . . . . . . . . . . .77

DiGiornio Cheese-Stuffed Crust,
　　Pepperoni Pizza . . . . . . . . . . . . . . . . . . . . . . . .79

## POULTRY

Arby's Prime-Cut Chicken Tenders with Chopped
　　Side Salad. . . . . . . . . . . . . . . . . . . . . . . . . . . .29

Boston Market Chicken Breast with Garlic Dill
　　New Potatoes and Chicken Tortilla Soup . . . .37

has been truly eye-opening. I learned so much from you about the special consequences of sugar for women that it literally shaped my mission in life. Being invited to participate in your PBS special was a dream come true.

To Dr. Andrew Weil—your continued support over the years has meant so much. More than any other M.D. in the public eye, your pursuit of a more integrative approach to health is exactly the message our society needs in these dire times.

Thank you to my entire group of invaluable health experts: Dr. Mehmet Oz, Dr. David Katz, Dr. James Novak, Dr. Terry Grossman, Dr. Ray Kurzweil, Dr. Nicholas Perricone, and Gary Taubes. I'm fortunate to have such renowned experts as mentors and friends.

A very special thanks to my friends and partners in media, who have been so critical in spreading this vital message: Rachael Ray, Abra Potkin, Janet Annino, John Redmann, Terence Noonan, Ginnie Roeglin, Anita Thompson, David Fuller, Tim Talevish, Maggie Jacqua, Beth Weissman, Scott Eason, Al Roker, Mark Victor, Bill Getty, Joy Behar, Thomas Walter, Priscilla Totten, Terry Wood, Maggie Barnes, Loren Nancarrow, Leslie Marcus, and Richard Heller.

To my amazing clients—you inspired me to believe that each and every person has the innate ability to seize the day and reach for the life of his or her dreams. A very special thanks to Amber Allen-Sauer, who didn't stop at just helping herself. Your giving nature and passion for spreading this message is exactly the kind of enthusiasm that drives positive change in our world. (Be sure to check out Amber's blog: **MeandJorge.com.**)

I'd like to also thank my good friends for their support this past year: Lisa Sharkey, Joe Boleware, Jeff Craig, Bo Bortner, Rich Segal, Lauri Stock, Dr. Bob Hirsch, Suze Orman, Bob Wietrak, Mary-Ellen Keating, Richard Galanti, Debbie Ford, Pennie Ianniciello, Mike Koenings, Jay Robb, Frank Kern, Chris Hendrickson, Anthony Robbins, Eben Pagan, Elliot Bisnow, Suzanne Somers, and Wayne Dyer.

Finally, I am tremendously grateful to my dearest friend, Heather Cruise, a beautiful and understanding woman with whom I share two amazing sons. Thank you for all your love, support, and belief for so many years. The best is yet to come. I love you very much, forever.

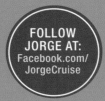

# About the Author

**JORGE CRUISE** is the #1 *New York Times* best-selling fitness author of over 20 diet and fitness books in over 16 languages. He is a contributor to *The Dr. Oz Show, Steve Harvey, Good Morning America*, the *Today* show, the *Rachael Ray Show*, EXTRA TV, Huffington Post, *First for Women Magazine,* and the *Costco Connection.*

Jorge received his bachelor's degree from the University of California, San Diego (UCSD); and has fitness credentials from the Cooper Institute for Aerobics Research, the American College of Sports Medicine (ACSM), and the American Council on Exercise (ACE).

To find out more about Jorge, visit **JorgeCruise .com.**

We hope you enjoyed this Hay House book. If you'd like to receive our online catalog featuring additional information on Hay House books and products, or if you'd like to find out more about the Hay Foundation, please contact:

Hay House, Inc., P.O. Box 5100, Carlsbad, CA 92018-5100
(760) 431-7695 or (800) 654-5126
(760) 431-6948 (fax) or (800) 650-5115 (fax)
www.hayhouse.com® • www.hayfoundation.org

• • •

**Published and distributed in Australia by:**
Hay House Australia Pty. Ltd., 18/36 Ralph St., Alexandria NSW 2015 •
*Phone:* 612-9669-4299 • *Fax:* 612-9669-4144 • www.hayhouse.com.au

**Published and distributed in the United Kingdom by:**
Hay House UK, Ltd., Astley House, 33 Notting Hill Gate, London W11 3JQ
*Phone:* 44-20-3675-2450 • *Fax:* 44-20-3675-2451 • www.hayhouse.co.uk

**Published and distributed in the Republic of South Africa by:**
Hay House SA (Pty), Ltd., P.O. Box 990, Witkoppen 2068
info@hayhouse.co.za

**Published in India by:**
Hay House Publishers India, Muskaan Complex, Plot No. 3, B-2,
Vasant Kunj, New Delhi 110 070 • *Phone:* 91-11-4176-1620
*Fax:* 91-11-4176-1630 • www.hayhouse.co.in

**Distributed in Canada by:**
Raincoast Books, 2440 Viking Way, Richmond, B.C. V6V 1N2
*Phone:* 1-800-663-5714 • *Fax:* 1-800-565-3770 • www.raincoast.com

• • •

**Take Your Soul on a Vacation**

Visit www.HealYourLife.com® to regroup, recharge, and reconnect with your own magnificence. Featuring blogs, mind-body-spirit news, and life-changing wisdom from Louise Hay and friends.